THE ACTUALLY PRETTY GOOD BABY

A parent-tested guide for moms who want to breastfeed *and* sleep through the night

SUSAN VUKADINOVIC

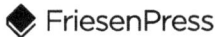
FriesenPress

One Printers Way
Altona, MB R0G 0B0
Canada

www.friesenpress.com

Copyright © 2023 by Susan Vukadinovic
First Edition — 2023

This book is designed to provide accurate information on the subject matter covered. It is sold with the understanding that neither the author nor the publisher are engaged in rendering psychological, medical, legal or other professional advice or services.

All children are unique and this book is not intended to substitute for the diagnostic expertise and medical advice of a qualified physician, whom readers should always consult when a child shows any sign of illness or unusual behaviour, as well as before beginning any sleep program or breastfeeding approach—to verify that the plan is acceptable for a particular child.

The author and publisher specifically disclaim all responsibility for any liability, loss or risk, personal or otherwise, which is incurred as a consequence, directly or indirectly, of the use and application of any of the contents of this book. Readers are strongly encouraged to use their own judgment in their parenting decisions.

Edited by Emily Donaldson
Cover design and illustrations by Kimberly Glyder
Author image by Janet Pliszka

All rights reserved. No part of this publication may be reproduced in any form, or by any means, electronic or mechanical, including photocopying, recording, or any information browsing, storage, or retrieval system, without permission in writing from FriesenPress.

ISBN
978-1-03-918077-2 (Hardcover)
978-1-03-918076-5 (Paperback)
978-1-03-918078-9 (eBook)

1. FAMILY & RELATIONSHIPS/LIFE STAGES/INFANTS & TODDLERS

Distributed to the trade by The Ingram Book Company

Author's Note:

For information on special discounts for bulk purchases, promotions and fundraising, or to get your very own copy of the black bean gruel recipe mentioned on page 268, please contact susanvukadinovic@gmail.com.

I have relied on many different sources for this book, and I have done my best to fact check and to trace the ownership of copyright material. In the event that material is incorrect or has been used without proper permission, I welcome information enabling me to rectify any oversights.

I also welcome information enabling me to make the black bean gruel recipe more palatable for my children. They're adamant that black bean gruel is an oversight that desperately needs to be rectified.

Susan Vukadinovic

TABLE OF CONTENTS

Introduction	vii
About This Book	ix
Part I: The Eight Operating Basics	**1**
Chapter 1: All You Need is Love	3
Part II: Your Step-By-Step Guide from Pregnancy to Age 3	**9**
Chapter 2: Pregnancy	11
Chapter 3: The Birth Day	13
Chapter 4: Day 2 and Day 3	29
Chapter 5: First Two Weeks	39
Chapter 6: Day 14 to Day 40	57
Chapter 7: Week 6 to Week 12	79
Chapter 8: Three Months Old	111
Chapter 9: Months Four and Five	119
Chapter 10: Six Months Old	143
Chapter 11: Months 7 to 11	155
Chapter 12: Months 12 to 15	165
Chapter 13: Months 16 to 24	189
Chapter 14: Months 24 to 36	203
Part III: Troubleshooting	**219**
Chapter 15: Formula	221
Chapter 16: Breastmilk	225
Chapter 17: Sleep	247
Chapter 18: The Ten Basics of Bed-Sharing	257
Chapter 19: The Twelve Most Frequently Asked Questions	261
Chapter 20: The Last Word	269
Resources Used & Recommended	**271**

INTRODUCTION

When I was pregnant with my first child, several friends, family members and co-workers shared this advice: It's best to introduce a bottle right from the start. Just in case. After all, despite *wanting* to breastfeed, many first-time moms find it hard to make enough milk. Plus, they claimed, a bottle would help with sleep-training.

(*Got it. Can of formula: stocked.*)

But then, shortly before my baby arrived, I found kindred spirits in the attachment-parenting crowd and my *new* new-mom posse had a different story to tell. They told me that with help and support most moms produce an ample supply of breastmilk; that it doesn't dry up on its own.

(*Okay, then. Can of formula: tossed.*)

But my new friends also said that anyone who suggests their baby slept through the night at two months of age was telling a tall tale. What's more, they claimed, sleep-training could sever the mother-child bond, so it was best to nurse baby throughout the night for as long as possible. Just in case.

(*Yikes!*)

For the first couple of years of motherhood, I muddled through, enjoying coffee and playdates with my separate groups of mom friends while navigating between their competing views. I breastfed like an attachment parent and I sleep-trained like a mom who goes out on date nights, and it never occurred to me that anyone else was doing both, too.

But then, a turning point.

Right around the time my second child was learning to crawl, I completed accreditation as a breastfeeding helper and I began facilitating workshops for new and expectant mothers. Over the next few years, through hundreds of conversations, I noticed a pattern that echoed the experiences of my closest friends: moms who figured out how to breastfeed often struggled to get their children to sleep, while moms who figured out how to sleep-train often struggled to keep breastfeeding.

It doesn't have to be this way.

By weaving together our collective momma wisdom, I've discovered—as have countless moms at my workshops—that it's possible to breastfeed *and* get a good night's sleep. You don't have to pick one or the other. You can do both!

This ultimate beginner's guide to babycare will show you how.

ABOUT THIS BOOK

It's a parent-tested approach.

Because I'm truly passionate about helping new moms, I've thoroughly tested the material in this book. You see, I started making tip sheets for the moms who attended my prenatal and new-baby workshops back in 2011, and the moms who came back month after month always let me know if something in those sheets didn't quite ring true. I would immediately incorporate the feedback I received, which made the tip sheets better, more accurate. Eventually, parents began asking me for the whole series, and it dawned on me: I had enough mom-tested and mom-approved tips and tricks to fill a whole book.

It takes a village to raise a child, and it took a community of parents to vet this book. That's why I call it a parent-tested approach.

It's a parent-tested approach and, yes, it works.

Everything I know about breastfeeding and baby sleep and babycare I've learned from listening to the only voices that really matter: mommas just like you. When a new mom pipes up at a workshop and tells other new moms, You've just *got* to try such and such, she's usually right. It's amazing.

Over the course of hundreds of heartfelt conversations, I've heard which babycare approaches and resources moms swear by, and which ones fall a little flat. I've figured out which stuff mommas need to know in advance, and what they have no trouble figuring out by themselves. And I've discovered that some questions come up over and over again, while others I've been trained to answer never come up at all.

Listening to and learning from the mommas at my workshops has helped me understand that there are simple, easy ways to navigate the baby years. There's a playbook for a well-fed, well-rested, contented baby, and the mommas who've been following it all along are swearing by the results.

This isn't really a parenting book.

I mean, I know you probably found this book in the parenting section of your favourite bookstore, which is where it should be, but this is actually a *babycare* book. So what's the difference between babycare and parenting?

I define *babycare* as the tactics and techniques used to care for a baby. Babycare covers the basics.

Everything beyond the basics qualifies as parenting. It's where the *magic* happens. But while I love magic, I'm no magician. I don't know the secret to better parenting. My shtick is babycare: pure and simple.

"There is no recipe for parenting."
"What works for one parent might not work for another."

These are sentences you'll find on virtually every parenting website, blog, podcast, or Twitter account. You'll even find them in most parenting books.

And I wholeheartedly agree. It would be futile to try to break *parenting* down into a set of easy-to-follow, one-size-fits-all instructions, because there truly is no one right way to parent.

And yet, shocking as it may sound: There actually *is* a recipe for babycare.

Unlike with parenting, it actually *is* possible (and helpful) to break babycare down into a set of easy-to-follow, one-size-fits-most instructions because the mechanics behind early breastfeeding, sleeping, diapering, and play are so universal. Once the basics are covered, you can parent any way you like.

It's a "how to," not a "how come?"

To keep this book as short as possible, while still covering the basics, I've focused on *what* to do, instead of *why* you should do it.

But if you're keen to learn more about any of the topics I cover, have a look at the recommended reading listed in the Resources section near the end.

Alternatively, you can hop on the internet bus and keep going until you find the right stop. Every single concept I bring up in this book is explained in greater detail in a blog or in an online, open-source academic journal or on a dedicated website. I'm talking pictures, background information, comprehensive explanations, research citations—the works—all available at your fingertips and all accessible for free on the good ol' worldwide web.

Right about now you may be thinking, *Why'd I shell out good money when I could've found everything I need to know on my smartphone? (For free!)*

I have an answer for that.

You see, the internet can be useful when it comes to problem solving, but it's less useful for new parents who want to avoid those problems in the first place. If parents google, "Is it normal that my three-month-old baby will only sleep in my arms?" they'll find out that it *is* normal. What they won't learn is that there are things they could have done early on to avoid this situation altogether. The answer to another common question—"Is it normal for breastmilk to dry up on its own at eight weeks?"—is, again, Yes. But there are things mom and dad[1] could have been doing from Day 1 to prevent it from happening. New parents can't google the questions that they don't know they should be googling. You don't know what you don't know.

Another reason you get good value learning about babycare from a book: a book is exactly the right length. The internet is both too long and too short to be helpful when it comes to the basics.

Here's what I mean when I say the internet is too long: This babycare book contains several hundred pages, which is long enough, but the internet is like a seven-billion-page babycare book. It's true. I just entered "how to care for a baby" into Google, and that's how many hits I got. It's out there, but you'll never get through it all.

At the same time, the internet is also too short. There are countless tweets, blogs, and 700-word articles available online and through social media, and most are smart and well written, but they're all—every one—constrained by the scariest four letters on the internet: TL;DR. *Too long; didn't read.*

Some aspects of babycare need more than 280 characters to be explained properly. If you're going to get into the nuances of breastfeeding or sleep, sometimes you need length. I'm sharing what I know about babycare in an old-timey book format because it's the *complete* package of information that's of value. As anyone who's tried to assemble Ikea furniture knows, you need more than sheer motivation to put it all together. You need to read the instructions. And it helps to read *all* the instructions—not just some of them.

---

1 When I use the words "mom" or "dad" throughout this book, I'm just using shorthand. What I really mean is: single and partnered parents of any gender. And when I say "parent," I also use that term broadly. I include all adults who play a primary role in caring for a baby, including biological parents, stepparents, grandparents, foster parents, guardians, aunties, uncles, and the like. I have warmth in my heart for everyone who has embarked on an adventure in parenting. Welcome to the tribe of mommas, whatever your many other identities might be!

Great minds think alike. Fools seldom differ.

There are contradictions in this book.

So as you're reading along you may stop and think, "Wait, didn't she just say the exact opposite thing a few pages back?"

Yes, I probably did, because a lot of baby and toddler care is based on contradictory concepts, like:

> Do nurse your baby to sleep. But there's no need to nurse your baby until he's asleep.
>
> Be present. But don't hover.
>
> Be child-led. But don't be child-centred.
>
> Share everything. Don't share.

The tricky thing is that, with all of these examples, *both* statements are correct. It all depends on the timing. Sometimes one applies to the newborn stage while the opposite applies to a toddler. Or sometimes one applies in most circumstances, but the opposite is an exception that applies only during a brief training stage.

This is why I've chosen to use a chronological, stage-by-stage approach in this book. Figuring out how to square conflicting advice is challenging for new parents, but it's a little easier when you know *when* to apply a nugget of wisdom. Often when parents struggle with a certain aspect of sleeping or feeding, it's because they heard about a good approach to try, but missed the window of opportunity in which to try it. Timing can make all the difference.

What makes this babycare book different?

What makes this book different from other babycare books is the combination of what I have woven in and what I have left out.

When I ran my prenatal and new-baby workshops, I often recommended books. Naturally, I couldn't recommend babycare books without reading them first, so I read about three dozen or so. I took a deep dive and, although a lot of what I read was very good,

I found a gap between what mommas were looking for and what the market was offering. I noticed that some books provided accurate information about breastfeeding, but these tended to be attachment-parenting books that scared moms away from taking back the night through sleep-training. Other books provided accurate information about sleep-training, but these tended to conflate providing accurate information about breastfeeding with creating pressure to breastfeed.

I was forever saying things like, "This book is a great resource for the breastfeeding issue you just raised, but ignore what it says about sleep because it could send you down a rabbit hole."

Or, "This book is super helpful when it comes to the sleeping challenge you talked about today, but be aware that some of the things it says about breastfeeding are a little outdated."

There simply wasn't a babycare book that accurately explained what it would take to get baby to breastfeed *and* sleep through the night.

I wrote this book for you—yes, *you*—because I think you might be just like me and the mommas at my workshops, and you want to do both, too: breastfeed *and* sleep. You *can* do both.

PART I:

THE EIGHT OPERATING BASICS

CHAPTER 1:

All You Need is Love

You've made a bold move. You're starting a family. *That's fantastic*! I am truly excited for you.

Before we dive into the step-by-step instructions, let's go over the eight operating basics for your brand-new baby. These are the hard-and-fast rules that apply regardless of where you're at in the newborn-to-toddler years.

Rule #1: All you need is love.[2]

The reason most kids turn out all right, no matter how they're raised, is because they have a flawed parent who is absolutely besotted with them. When you get right down to it, what small children need

---

2   **Source:** Virtually anything written by Gabor Maté.
    Oh, and the Beatles, obviously.
    And Urie Bronfenbrenner, Benjamin Spock, John Bowlby, Mary Ainsworth, Patricia Crittenden, Mary Main, Brené Brown, Nicole Letourneau, and Dolly Parton.
    Although, really, Saints Augustine, Aquinas, and Paul came up with it first…
    You know what, forget sources. We're talking common knowledge here, people. All you need is love.

most from their parents is sustained, loving attention. They need our deepest affection.

This is why, by the time they're school-aged, you can't tell which kids were breastfed and which ones were nourished with formula. You can't tell which kids were sleep-trained and which ones shared a bed with mom and dad at night. They all seem more or less the same—sometimes happy, sometimes sulky, sometimes warmly attached, and sometimes fiercely independent—but with an undercurrent of resilience that will help most of them get through whatever life throws their way.

That resilience comes from an abundance of love.

Rule #2: Take it easy.

Taking it easy doesn't mean always doing what's easiest at any given moment. When it comes to raising a baby, it often seems like making your life easier in the long run means doing something right now that isn't easy at all.

In the long run you probably want a well-rested, less cranky child. Tonight, this might mean going through the pain of sleep-training.

In the long run you might want to try breastfeeding. Today, this could mean some marathon nursing to establish breastmilk supply.

Some parenting philosophies send parents down rabbit holes by encouraging them to do what's "most natural" for baby or what's "best" for baby or what will keep baby "happiest." Not that there's anything wrong with trying to do what's "most natural" or "best" for your baby. Happiness isn't a bad aim, either.

But keep in mind that the parent next door who's not fussed about "natural" or "best" will end up with a seven-year-old who's just as well attached and adjusted as the child whose aspirational parents earnestly tried to do everything right.

Going back to Rule #1: Sustained, loving attention is an incredibly important part of raising healthy, happy children. So much so that almost nothing else you do will create as much of an appreciable difference in how they turn out.

So you might as well make the parenting journey easy on *yourself*.

Rule #3: Never let baby cry. Your child will carry the trauma for life.

There was a period when Western society held a misguided notion that babies should be left to cry, because this would somehow exercise their lungs, or build greater independence, or show them who's boss early on. "Don't pick him up. It's good for him to cry."

But then, in 1946, Dr. Benjamin Spock published *The Common Sense Book of Baby and Child Care*, which changed the dominant approach to child care in North America. The book re-introduced a notion that our great-great-great-grandmothers would have found obvious: If a baby is crying, pick him up. In his initially controversial book, which eventually sold 50 million copies and influenced an entire generation of parents, Dr. Spock pushed back against early-20th-century expert advice that said showing children affection would spoil them.

Dr. Spock's common-sense approach has stood the test of time. Leaving a baby to cry simultaneously breaks Rules #1 and #2. No one enjoys hearing a crying baby's squalls. And ignoring your child's grief goes against what your momma heart tells you to do. Plus, leaving your baby to cry doesn't build independence. Nor will it show your baby who's boss.

The babies whose needs are immediately met are the ones who end up gurgling and cooing adoringly at everyone and who have lovely, calm dispositions.

So, never, ever let your baby cry.

Rule #4: It's perfectly fine to let baby cry right now. Don't worry about it. Baby will be fine.

This is where parenting is more art than science. If you figure out the sweet spot where Rules #3 and #4 can simultaneously be true in a non-parallel universe, then you'll totally ace this baby-raising gig.

Rule #5. Sometimes, maybe, just give it a minute.

Good things come to those who wait. The frantically rooting newborn will latch. The crying baby will fall asleep. The lost toddler will round the corner of the next aisle in the grocery store and run towards you with a smile. When the *All* *Systems* *Fail* sign is frantically flashing, sometimes it helps to hit the pause button and take a deep breath.

    Breathe.

Rule #6. Listen to your instincts. Except when your instincts are wrong.

On the one hand, you need to trust your mom gut. You know better than anyone what your baby needs.

On the other hand, be open to the possibility that your instincts could be woefully wrong. Your instincts might say, "Maybe TikTok knows more than my doctor" (it doesn't), or, "Maybe my baby is allergic to tomatoes" (he isn't). If you suspect your mom gut is being irrational, feel free to fall back on good ol' trusty science.

Ah, yes. Science.

Individual studies can contradict each other, but on balance, over time, the knowledge we gain through systematic study is really quite reliable.

Rule #7. Do a good job. A good-enough job.

As long as you're trying your hardest, and you're having fun doing it, don't let perfect be the enemy of good. The occasional late bedtime, burnt casserole, or sugary snack won't destroy *everything.*

Anytime you're feeling inadequate, take comfort in the fact that billions of amateurs have botched the parenting gig before you. We all take turns being highly underprepared or needlessly overwhelmed.

You're human like the rest of us.

Rule #8. Do what works for you.

Many parenting books imply that unless you follow the author's instructions, you'll damage your child forever. Follow the strictures of attachment parenting, or your child will be a sullen, sodden, weepy mess. Sleep-train or your child's IQ will be stunted. Take a vacation with just your partner, or your child will never leave your side long enough to start kindergarten.

Let me be very clear: If you don't follow all the steps in this book, *nothing bad will happen.*

This book wasn't written to help make you a perfect parent. Nor will it help you raise a perfect baby.

This play-by-play guide was written with a single purpose: to make the baby-raising stage as easy as possible for mom and dad. And because the content of this book is purely intended to make your life easier, there's no foul if you decide to take a pass on any of it. You get to make the final call on what to feed your baby and when to wean him and how to raise him.

Do what works for you, and leave the rest behind.

PART II:

YOUR STEP-BY-STEP GUIDE FROM PREGNANCY TO AGE 3

CHAPTER 2:

Pregnancy

Many moms read about pregnancy and the birthing process while they're expecting. The plan is to learn about babies…later.

The thing is: there are specific things you can do in the first minutes and hours after birth that will make your new adventure in parenting run more smoothly. And trust me, you won't be picking up a babycare book mere minutes after delivering your baby. You'll have other, more important things on your mind.

So, I recommend you read the next few chapters of this book now, *before* baby arrives, to find out how you're going to lay down your prolactin receptors.

Prolactin receptors? Whaaaat?!

Yeah.
It helps to know what's coming.

CHAPTER 3:

The Birth Day

If you want to start at the beginning, which seems like a very good place to start, then this is where our adventure begins: Your baby's birth day. Girl, it's *your* Mother's Day!

First thing's first: Snuggle up, skin-to-skin.

Your baby just spent nine months or so in your womb. Right after birth, his natural habitat is still your body. So, shortly after he arrives, take your top off (you just gave birth, so semi-nudity isn't going to feel like a big deal). Then snuggle together, skin-to-skin.

Touch is the most meaningful sensation for your infant. Until just a few minutes ago, your baby had spent his entire existence floating weightlessly in his aquatic cocoon. Unable to speak, unable to smell, hearing only muffled sounds and seeing only changes in light, your new baby's chief connection to the world around him had been made through his sense of touch. In the moments after birth, your skin's warmth, texture, motion, and gravitational pull all speak to him in a language he's already learned. You are his wilderness and he's safe here.

If you're not able to hold baby skin-to-skin during the first hour or two after birth, then your partner or other family members can take on this role.

The goal of raising children isn't to draw them closer, but to ultimately set them free. But not at Step 1. Right now, pull him in.

Next: Give baby a gentle towel rub.

Vernix Caseosa is a white, slippery, cream-cheese-like substance found on baby's skin at birth. It provides waterproofing for baby in utero and appears to play a role in helping his skin transition from the high-humidity surroundings found in the uterus to the much lower humidity levels found in, say, a prairie hospital in March. When a newborn receives a simple towel rub instead of a thorough washing, the vernix will absorb into his skin in the first 24 to 48 hours after birth.

While you can ask your birthing team to gently use a cloth or towel to wipe off traces of blood and amniotic fluid (either before they hand him over for his first cuddle or while he's lying on your, or your partner's, chest), the World Health Organization recommends delaying your baby's first water-immersion or sponge bath for at least six hours post-partum. Some experts even recommend waiting several days. Either way, bathing doesn't need to be the first priority right after birth.

Before baby arrives, talk to your birthing team about their plans for bathing baby and examining baby's health, and how these things can be incorporated around skin-to-skin cuddle time as soon as possible after birth.

Now lean back in a reclined position and place your baby "tummy-to-mommy."

Once you've had a chance to catch your breath after giving birth, shimmy your body into a reclined position. (Reclined is partway between fully upright and lying down.)

Most newborn babies prefer to be snuggled in a **vertical** hold against momma, at least <u>for the first hour or so</u>, rather than held in a horizontal, sideways cradle hold. A vertical position means your baby is lying flat on your bare tummy, with his body lined up in the *same* direction as your body. Gently move his arms out of the way so his chest is flat against your own. If you like, you can cover yourself and baby with a light blanket for warmth.

It's not quite time to try breastfeeding yet, but this is a great position to breastfeed in if you are planning to do so. Newborn babies, like newborn kittens and puppies, are "tummy feeders," which means they nurse best when their bare tummies are touching mom's skin.

But hold on. Take it easy. As I said before, you're not trying to latch on your baby just yet. Right now, you're just relaxing in a reclined, skin-to-skin position and cuddling your new baby.

Even if you're not planning to breastfeed, your baby will still like it here. He can hear your heartbeat—just like he did in the womb. The skin-to-skin contact will keep your baby calm and stabilize his body temperature. And hearing and feeling the rise and fall of your inhalations and exhalations while lying on your chest will help him organize his own breathing.

Even mommas who've had a cesarean section are usually able to hold their babies in this position quite soon after birth.

Take a good look at your baby.

What an absolute miracle!

For your baby's first half hour or so of life, he'll likely alternate between several minutes of being completely relaxed and not moving and then several minutes of activity where he moves his head, mouth, eyes, and shoulders. During the periods where he's active, you may notice that he's beginning to make sucking movements and rooting with his mouth.

There's nothing special you need to do or not do at this point. If you can, take your time and just enjoy your new baby.

There was a time when mommas were told to try breastfeeding right after birth and to tickle baby's lips with the nipple, but this can interfere with baby's instincts and make everyone feel frustrated.

(If your baby is medically vulnerable, your health professionals may determine that he needs to be encouraged to begin latching faster. If this happens, just roll with it. A baby with health challenges needs medical advice. But if your baby is in good health, breastfeeding will be easier if you don't rush into trying to latch your baby for that first half hour or so.)

Between 20 and 40 minutes after birth, your baby will start pushing against your body with his feet and arms. He'll use these primitive neonatal reflexes to make crab-like crawling movements that get him closer to the breast and nipple.

Again, if your baby is not medically vulnerable, there's nothing special you need to do or not do at this point. Trust yourself to instinctively feel how much help to give your baby.

Take it all in.

Take your time…

For the next half hour, baby will familiarize himself with the breast and nipple. His hands may touch and massage the breast. He may bob his head. He may touch the nipple with his mouth or tongue (but not quite latch on).

Finally, about <u>an hour</u> after his birth, your baby will self-attach to the nipple and suckle.

Make your breast easier to latch onto.

If you need to help your baby latch on (either because a medical vulnerability means health professionals want you to begin nursing faster, or because it's been more than an hour since his birth and your baby seems to be struggling with latching on his own), a trick that often works is to make the breast easier to latch onto by using your chicken wing to make a hamburger. Let me explain.

Decide which breast you'd like to try nursing with first. Whichever you choose, stick out your elbow on that side and form a "chicken wing."

Now you're going to use the hand on your chicken-wing arm to shape your breast like a hamburger. You do this by placing your thumb on top of your breast, away from the areola (the dark area around your nipple), and placing your remaining four fingers underneath your breast.

Think about how you hold a hamburger—thumb on one side and the rest of the fingers on the other side, **but reversed**.

Think about how you hold a hamburger when you bring it to your mouth—it's horizontal, not vertical. Whichever angle your baby is positioned in when you bring him to your breast, you'll have to line up your breast—aka the hamburger—so it's horizontal to his mouth.

Think about the strength you use to do this. You're not trying to squeeze the bun into a squishy mess. Use a firm but gentle grip.

Are you picturing it?[3]

Going one step at a time, bring baby into position...

Use your free arm (and, if you like, the helping hands of your partner, nurse, or midwife) to position your baby.

It doesn't matter which direction your baby is facing, as long as you're both comfortable. For starters, just focus on getting baby's bare chest against your bare body, regardless of whether he's lying on your tummy or against your side.

Okay, let's do a bit more adjusting: face your baby toward your breast (not the ceiling).

Some newborns nurse better if their feet are touching or pushing against momma's body, or a solid object (like your mattress), so maybe check if he's got a "foothold" available.

---

[3] If not, you'll find helpful resources, illustrations and videos if you google "breastfeeding" and "sandwich hold."

THE BIRTH DAY

One more thing: Your baby's ear, shoulder, and hip bone should be in a straight line. In other words, your baby's head shouldn't be twisted to the side. It's hard for a baby to swallow when his neck is twisted. Imagine eating an entire meal while looking over one of your shoulders.

We're good?[4]

Ok. Now, with your baby in position, wait for him to open his mouth as wide as a yawn… and… and…

Latch.

Figuring out how to latch a baby is a major part of Day 1. Even if mom is experienced, baby isn't. Then there are the additional complications of a very large nipple, a very tiny mouth, and baby's total lack of head control. It's easy to get frustrated.

If you're having a tough go of it, here's a little pep talk.

Hang in there. It's like learning to ride a bicycle.

Figuring out how to latch a baby is a messy, difficult process. It's not like studying for an exam.

It's more like learning to ride a bicycle. You can't really do it by reading instructions from a book. You need to get on, start pedalling, fall off, then keep getting on again every time you fall off. It's awkward, it doesn't work right away, but then eventually it all just sort of…clicks.

---

[4] If you need more help visualizing all of this, Dr. Suzanne Colson, a renowned expert on laidback breastfeeding, has an excellent website as well as a great book on the topic. I particularly recommend you google her two-minute video clip.
You could also check out this online excerpt from the classic book, *The Womanly Art of Breastfeeding*: lllc.ca/sites/default/files/Laid-back-bf_WAB.pdf. Better yet, run out and buy your own copy of *The Womanly Art of Breastfeeding*. It's a super helpful resource, and the more you learn about breastfeeding from different sources, the more comfortable and confident you'll be as a nursing momma.

So, don't overthink the latch—just try it. And then try it again. And then again.

Believe in yourself. You can do this. You really can.

Professional athletes talk about being in "the Zone"—that feeling they get in the heat of competition where things become effortless. Intuition takes over, all tension is released, and they can just "do" instead of "trying to do." You're trying to get into the Zone, too. And you'll get there. You will! It may be frustrating now, but once it clicks, you'll be able to latch your baby effortlessly.

Remember, your body and your baby's body are *designed* to make this happen.

Things still not gelling?

Seek help from someone who knows what they're doing.

This can be a health professional at the hospital where you gave birth, a midwife, a lactation consultant, or an experienced mother in any number of other settings.

If you didn't get the help you needed from the first person you asked, then ask another person and try their suggestions. Rinse. Repeat. Sometimes new moms have to ask more than one person for help before they find the person whose support works for them.

If six different health professionals have given you six different versions of how to get this baby to start nursing, instead of feeling annoyed, look on the bright side. Every breastfeeding experience is unique, so the more suggestions you get, the better your chances of finding the special trick that will work for **you** and *your* particular baby. To put it in engineering terms, it's like triangulation with two data points; all you need is one more input and everything will fall into place.

When it comes to a brand-new baby, nothing replaces one-on-one contact and discussion with actual human beings. No book, no internet site, no poster on a birthing-room wall will be as rich a resource as the community of moms and health professionals who will come by to visit with you or check on you on Day 1. Be open to their suggestions, even when they contradict each other.

Finally—a comfortable latch!

Once your baby has latched onto your breast, his mouth should be covering the nipple and as much of the areola as possible. A midwife, doula, or health professional may also look to see if there are sucking motions along baby's jawline.

If something doesn't feel right, unlatch and try again.

It's normal for latching to take several attempts. If something doesn't feel right and you want to unlatch, insert your finger in baby's mouth to break the suction. If you don't break the suction before unlatching your baby, you risk injuring your nipple.

This will be your baby's first experience using all five senses.

Advances in artificial intelligence are based, in part, on the concept of "machine learning," where computer systems use algorithms to identify patterns and make inferences without explicit instructions from a human programmer. But scientists know that humans are much more sophisticated at identifying patterns and making inferences than even the smartest AI device. That's because the human brain gets inputs from our sense of taste, smell, touch, sight, and hearing, and not just from our neurons firing the equivalent of binary-code zeros and ones.

The human brain is truly remarkable. We can spot patterns in our environment, and then we can use those patterns to make educated guesses about the world, and then we can build on these educated guesses to make imaginative leaps about what we could change, and then we can communicate our ideas to other humans and convince them to change things with us. Sometimes this works out for humanity and sometimes, well, not so much, but it's pretty cool that we have this ability. It's what makes us special.

And this pattern-making begins on Day 1. No machine could ever equal the magic that begins unfolding at the moment of his first feeding, when your baby first uses all five senses—taste, smell, touch, hearing, and sight—all at momma's breast, and all at the same time.

Now that your baby has started using all five of his senses to learn about his world, wait 'til you see the patterns he'll figure out and inferences he'll make in the next three years. You'll have such a clever baby, Momma!

Your plan for the rest of the day: Hang out.

You've got your first breastfeeding experience under your belt, so what's next?

More of the same! These early days of motherhood are a full-body experience, so plan to spend as much skin-to-skin time together as possible.

You can expect to have baby at your breast for around *eight* of his first 24 hours. But don't be a martyr. If you need a break, you can swaddle baby, put him in a bassinet, and get some shut-eye. Today, your main tasks are twofold: to take care of baby's needs *and* to take care of yourself as a brand-new momma.

Eight hours per day—but not all in one shift.

Think about it: eight hours of breastfeeding. If you worked before your baby arrived, imagine shifts that long.

Basically, this is your new job.

But rest assured: It's just for the first few days. After that, baby gets much more efficient at feeding and time spent at the breast goes down significantly week by week.

Another thing: Moms are more likely to have success breastfeeding if they're aware that newborns do *not* breastfeed at regular intervals (such as every two hours). Instead, newborn babies have a natural inclination to cluster their feedings together. Sometimes a newborn will breastfeed frequently for short periods—maybe a few minutes every hour. But other times a newborn will breastfeed for long stretches, even hours at a time. He's going to do it his own way until mother's milk becomes more abundant or "comes in." As long as the accumulated time at the breast is about eight hours over the first 24 hours after birth, though, it doesn't matter how he spaces out his nursings.

What does it mean for milk to "come in"?

Colostrum is the initial milk a woman produces midway through pregnancy and during the first few days after she delivers her baby. It's a thick, concentrated fluid, often golden in colour. Rich in nutrients, antibodies, and other protective factors, it's basically your baby's first superfood.

During the first 24 hours of nursing, your baby gets only about 30 mL (one ounce) of colostrum in total, spread out over all his feedings. In other words, you're going to spend this whole first day trying to figure out how to latch and breastfeed and 30 mL is all he's going to get. Most mommas can do this, even with that very awkward first day of feeding, because it's such a tiny amount.

There's a reason your body produces this minute volume of colostrum. Until just a few hours ago, your baby was being nourished by an umbilical cord, so it's going to take him a bit of time to get used to using his tiny mouth to eat and his tiny tummy to digest food. Your baby's stomach at birth is about the size of a cherry, so your early milk comes super concentrated so as not to overload that little tummy. And the small quantity of colostrum gives your baby a chance to get these new body parts working without being overwhelmed by a gush of milk. Remember: this baby *just* rolled off the assembly line!

Milk is said to have "come in" when the thick, golden colostrum is replaced by a thin, bluish fluid that your body produces in a significantly higher volume.

Waiting three to five days for milk to come in is typical.

Breastfed newborns can nurse in their sleep.

Babies tend to be very awake for the first two hours after birth, and then they take their first nap. After that first good nap, a newborn baby will frequently fall asleep at the breast.

If your baby falls asleep at your breast, you can just leave him there. As long as his lips haven't sleepily fallen away from your breast, this counts as "time at the breast" and will help bring in your milk.

Many people call this time together a "babymoon."
Back when arranged marriages were more common—when few people had the privilege of marrying for love—a honeymoon provided important time for a new couple to get to know one another.

You can think of your relationship with your new baby as an arranged marriage, too. Before today you'd never met, and yet here you are, forever linked. You've basically agreed to a sacred vow—to love and to cherish, to comfort and to hold, to feed and to clothe and to shelter and protect for as long as you both shall live. That's some heavy stuff.

Just as a honeymoon is meant to be a private affair, a babymoon also works best if mom and baby have a relatively private environment to begin their bonding. (And yes, I realize the word *babymoon* has been co-opted by Instagrammers to mean a couple's last trip before the birth of their first child. But stick with me here. The words *honeymoon* and *babymoon* were both conceived as a month of bonding, not a week of travel.)

This time to hang out with your baby is important. It's not just about feeding him and getting your milk to come in. It's also about giving yourself time to adjust to this brand-new business of mothering.

> A confession:
> Sometimes
> It can be hard to love a newborn baby.

On the one hand, your newborn is an amazing little miracle and you've been waiting for him in what has felt like forever!

On the other hand, you don't really know this little stranger, and you may not have much in common, yet.

And so as you gaze into the wrinkled, beet-red, prune face of this mewling infant you might experience rumbling, low-grade regret

THE BIRTH DAY 23

tinged with existential dread and ladled over with a visceral sense of foreboding that you're in for a world of trouble. *Everything was going fine. We just paid off a chunk of our mortgage. I finally got on permanent at work. Why did we add a baby to the mix? What have we *done*?*

Relax. Sit back. Bedding in for a babymoon and spending lots of time nursing skin-to-skin will give the two of you something to do while you gradually—leisurely—get to know one another. You might even enjoy these peaceful moments of downtime with your napping, nursing infant nestled in your arms.

But at some point, you'll have to put baby down, so you can sleep.

At some point in the first 24 hours, momma needs to sleep, too. When *you're* ready to sleep, Momma, you have four main options for where to put your baby:

- **Option 1:** Baby sleeps on a separate sleep surface in a separate room from you.

- **Option 2:** You and baby share a room, with the two of you sleeping on **separate** surfaces (for example, you in an adult bed and baby in a bassinet next to the adult bed).

- **Option 3:** You and baby share a room and also share the **same** sleep surface, with baby *next* to you.

- **Option 4:** You and baby share a room and also share the **same** sleep surface, with baby sleeping directly *on* your chest (or dad's chest when you collapse from exhaustion). In other words, this is the option where the whole tummy-to-mommy bit continues even when mommy is trying to sleep.

There are families who follow each of these paths, whether by conscious design or because they just fall into it. However, only two of these four options are good ones.

Let's eliminate Option 1, at least for nighttime sleep once you're home. For the first four to six months of a baby's life, a crib in a separate room is one of the less desirable places for him to sleep at night. It makes it harder to breastfeed, because you have to travel further, and it puts your baby at increased risk for sudden unexpected death in infancy.[5] For about the first half year of a baby's life, most pediatricians agree that the safest place for baby to sleep is in the same room as his mother.[6]

Option 2 is a good one. Sharing the same room but sleeping on separate surfaces is the nighttime sleep arrangement that seems to attract the least controversy.

Option 3 is also viable, despite having its share of detractors. Chapter 18 has more information about this option. Some families fully embrace bed-sharing, while others treat it as a non-starter. Different strokes for different folks.

Option 4 is the one that many families fall into and then discover, too late, that they've ended up with a nightmare scenario: a baby who flatly refuses to sleep anywhere but in the tender embrace of mom or dad. So then mom and dad start sleeping in shifts, subbing one another off like players on a hockey team. Exhaustion sets in, then irritability, resentment, recriminations, and rage. Anytime you hear a parent complain, "My baby will only nap if I'm holding him," you'll know they went with Option 4.

Let me be clear: *every* baby prefers to sleep in momma's arms.

Every baby.

Every time.

The difference between babies who can only sleep in arms and the babies who can sleep on other surfaces lies with mom and dad.

To avoid the perils of Option 4, parents have to navigate one of the many aspects of baby-raising where two mutually exclusive rules are simultaneously applicable in a non-parallel universe:

---

5   Medical professional are moving away from the term familiar to most people, SIDS, or Sudden Infant Death Syndrome.

6   If you're still in the hospital or birthing centre, then the nursery is a safe place too, because a nurse or other health professional will be watching your baby and will let you know if he's hungry.

THE BIRTH DAY

- **Rule #1:** Do let your baby sleep on momma.
- **Rule #2:** Never, ever let your baby sleep on momma.

Rule #1: Do let baby sleep on momma.

Taking a babymoon and keeping your baby tummy-to-mommy as much as possible is the most effective way to establish an adequate breastmilk supply. If your baby falls asleep at the breast, he's logging "nursing time," which will help bring in your milk. And if he's not at the breast, you can still absolutely let him sleep cuddled against you.

There's a beautiful poem by Ruth Hulburt Hamilton (1921-2018) called *Song for a Fifth Child*, which I had printed and hung on my fridge for a good five years when my children were at their littlest, and it ends with the line, "Babies don't keep." Oh, it's true, young Momma, babies don't keep! There are few things sweeter in this fleeting life than a newborn sleeping in his mother's embrace. So do let your baby sleep on you, Momma.

Rule #2: Never, ever let baby sleep on momma.

Never when momma is sleeping, that is. Your little baby is precious. But do you know who else is precious? You are! And don't sub in your partner as a sleep surface when you're ready to turn in. If momma's ready to sleep, and baby's ready to sleep, then the whole family has a natural opportunity to give baby the type of deep, restful slumber that comes when he doesn't have an adult's shifting, sweating body beneath him.

A newborn typically sleeps 16–17 hours in a 24-hour period, while an adult normally needs seven to eight hours of shut-eye each night. That 10-hour difference between your sleep needs and your baby's leaves plenty of time for your little jellybean to enjoy languorous, daytime slumbers in the arms of mom, dad, grandma, grandpa, and all the other people who love him. Try to carve out at least seven hours each day—preferably at night—when you can doze off without a baby snoozing on your chest.

The mommas at my workshops have shared over and over: Let baby sleep in your arms as much as you like when you're *awake*, but when *you're* ready to sleep, do your whole family a favour and put baby down on his own sleep surface.

Make a plan for nighttime feeds.

Newborns wake to feed frequently, throughout the day and night, and they need to be fed on demand. Some families assume that the best way to help a new mom is to divvy up the nighttime between her, the other parent, and possibly even grandparents or a night nanny.

That's fine if Plan A is to nourish baby with formula. But if mom plans to breastfeed, the challenges with this are two-fold.

First, research indicates that even if someone else is doing the feeding, moms still tend to wake up at night if their babies are within hearing range, as they're biologically programmed to do. And if dad or another caregiver is doing the feeding, that likely means bottles, which means baby needs to wait for the bottle to be prepared—and babies are *terrible* at waiting—which means everyone is fully awake by the time baby begins feeding.

With breastfeeding, on the other hand, not only is the food instantly available in just the right amount and at just the right temperature, it's also possible to feed baby while mom is in a light sleep. This is because your body releases the hormone oxytocin as you nurse, which helps you relax and feel drowsy.

The second challenge with splitting night-feeding duties is that even though it makes things easier for mom in the short term (sleep! beautiful, beautiful sleep!—assuming mom has picked a spot to spend the night out of earshot of her baby), in the long term, she'll struggle to breastfeed. Nighttime bottlefeeding is incompatible with establishing an adequate milk supply, because night nursing in the early weeks plays an important role in boosting a mother's milk-production hormones.

Alternating between bottlefeeding and breastfeeding also increases the likelihood that baby will stage a nursing strike and refuse the breast entirely in a few weeks. Receiving a bottle's flow is a lot less work than suckling at the breast. Your baby's no fool. Once he figures out that there *is* such a thing as a free lunch, there's no way he's going to breastfeed.

For many moms debating whether to split night feedings with other people in the early days, it comes down to this: the extra time and frustration that come with trying to resolve breastfeeding struggles down the road may not be worth the extra nighttime shut-eye right now.

The good news is that the most intense nighttime feeding phase takes place over the first 40 days or so of your baby's life. It feels like forever when you're in the middle of it, but it will come to an end, I swear.

So try not to think of it as *sacrificing* yourself to establish breastmilk supply, but rather as *investing* time now to have an easier go of things later on. You're not Mother Theresa in this scenario. You're Warren Buffett. Or like a junior stockbroker on Wall Street—the kind who puts in 60-hour workweeks on the trading floor and then retires at 40.

CHAPTER 4:

Day 2 and Day 3

We get a little older every day, Momma. Welcome to your baby's second day!

Weigh your baby.

Babies who are born to term (i.e., not premature) lose 7-10 percent of their birth weight in the first few days following birth. This is normal and expected.

But did you know that the intravenous fluids a mother receives during the last two hours of the birthing process can inflate her baby's birth weight?

If you received IV fluids during birth and baby's weight loss is greater than 10 percent, there's no need to panic—your baby's weight loss could be greater than 10 percent if he's shedding this excess fluid through urine. ***On its own***, a greater-than-10-percent weight loss isn't enough to warrant supplementing baby's diet with bottled milk.

Consider asking ask your healthcare professional to weigh baby when he's 24-hours old, especially if you received IV fluids during labour. This 24-hour weight can then be used as the baseline for weight-loss-percentage calculations.

Intravenous fluids account for weight loss *only* during the first day, so unexpectedly large weight loss after the 24-hour mark (and especially after the three-day point) requires careful monitoring by a health professional.[7] But if baby's weight loss is within the expected range using the 24-hour mark, you're probably good.

Take a babymoon.

On Day 2 and Day 3, you'll want to keep spending heaps of time in bed, skin-to-skin and tummy-to-mommy with your newborn, in a reclined position. Remember, skin-to-skin means that your baby is wearing nothing but a diaper as he cuddles against your body. Of course, babies also enjoy skin-to-skin cuddling with other family members, so your partner can take part in the babymoon, too.

There's a strong link between taking a babymoon and reaching your breastfeeding goals—whether that goal is to breastfeed for a day or breastfeed for a year. This is partly because cuddling skin-to-skin increases a mother's levels of prolactin—the hormone that produces breastmilk.

But babymoons aren't just for breastfeeding families. There are half a dozen reasons why taking a babymoon makes *everyone* feel good:

A babymoon gets your feet up.

During pregnancy your body stored extra fluids. After your baby's birth, this fluid may collect in your feet and ankles for a few weeks. You'll eventually get rid of it by passing urine, but—until that happens—it helps if you're reclining with your feet up.

---

[7] Source: (1) Systematic Review: Noel-Weiss, J., et al. "Physiological weight loss in the breastfed neonate: A systematic review." *Open Medicine,* Vol 2, No 4 (2008); and (2) Noel-Weiss, J., et al. "An observational study of associations among maternal fluids during parturition, neonatal output, and breastfed newborn weight loss." *International Breastfeeding Journal,* Vol 6, No 9 (2011).

A babymoon forces you to take time for yourself.

There's a link between postpartum depression and trying to take on too much, too soon. By sitting around in bed, you may find it easier to clear your schedule, take in just one thing at a time, and slowly grow confidence in your new role as a mother.

It positions your baby more comfortably for reflux.

Babies are born with immature sphincter muscles, which essentially act as a doorway to the stomach. These immature sphincter muscles don't always close completely, allowing milk and stomach acid to come back up the esophagus—the muscular tube that connects throat to stomach. The result is spit-up or reflux. Although spit-up generally isn't harmful for your baby, it's unpleasant.

When moms or dads lean back in a reclined position, they'll naturally hold baby upright against their chest, which helps a newborn deal with reflux more comfortably. Think of it this way: If some of what you just ate was burbling back up into your mouth, would you rather be upright, facing forward, or lying on your back?

A babymoon counts as "tummy time" for your newborn.

Healthcare professionals recommend daily tummy time so your baby doesn't develop a flat area on his head. Time spent lying "tummy-to-mommy" counts towards this tummy time.

Human skull bones are soft until about 12 months of age. As a result, flat areas on the head can develop very quickly. Infants who spend too much time lying on their backs looking straight up may develop a flat area on the back of the head (brachycephaly). Infants who always lie with their heads turned to one side may develop flatness only on one side of the head (plagiocephaly), which can lead to changes in facial symmetry. While neither brachycephaly nor plagiocephaly will affect a baby's mental or physical development, the changes to his appearance can be permanent.

A babymoon helps regulate your baby's temperature.

Another benefit of skin-to-skin cuddling is that your body becomes aware of your baby's temperature. If your baby is too cool or too warm, your body temperature will rise or fall by one or two degrees to warm up or cool him down. Really! Our bodies are amazing.

A babymoon makes your baby feel good, too.

A skin-to-skin cuddle increases the release of oxytocin in moms and dads. Oxytocin is a hormone that reduces stress and helps bond a baby to his parents. A newborn is also calmer when he can hear mom's or dad's heartbeat and feel his parents' warmth. Bottom line: babies like cuddles.

Offer both breasts at each feeding.

Your baby was born with a stomach the size of a cherry, but by Day 3 it's grown to the size of a ping pong ball. However, because human milk rarely comes in by Day 3, despite spending lots of time at your breast, chances are that your baby still isn't getting very much to eat. This is normal and expected.

Offer both breasts at each feeding, especially in these early days, but don't worry about how frequently you're switching from breast to breast. Just switch when you feel like it. *Offer* both breasts at each feed, but let your baby decide if he wants the second side.

Getting your baby to sleep and getting your baby to eat are one and the same at this stage.

Newborns sleep around 16–17 hours total each day.

While newborns sleep a lot, their longest single sleep period may only be around four or five hours. And while mom would prefer this longest sleep period to occur at night, during the newborn stage it can happen at any point during the 24-hour day.

The second night is when many newborns really wake up!

Frequent night feedings are common for newborn babies, starting on the second night. Newborns at this stage tend to breastfeed the **least** from **3 to 9 am**. Feeding frequency then *increases* throughout the day, with several feedings between **9 pm and 3 am**. (3 am! Sorry.) Being awake this late is exhausting, but keep in mind that it's normal newborn behaviour, and this phase will pass very soon.

On Night 2 and Night 3, if your baby wants to nurse until 3 or 4 am, everything will go a lot smoother if you draw on your inner reserves and just do it. Your baby *will* eventually fall asleep tonight, I promise, even if it's in the middle of the night. At that point you can finally get some rest, too, and dream about the day when this night nursing will end. It's coming!

Newborns sometimes bob on and off the breast.

If your newborn is bobbing on and off the breast on Day 2 and Day 3, rest assured this is normal. On the second day, or night, many moms find that baby nurses for a bit, then goes to sleep. As soon as you take him off to put him in his bassinet he cries again and starts rooting around. So you latch him again. And then he unlatches. This can go on for hours.

A lot of moms become convinced this is because their milk isn't in yet and their baby is starving. But the reality is that babies tend to bob on and off on Day 2 or Night 2 even when a mom's milk comes in early.

Again, this is where taking a babymoon can be helpful. Mothers who don't hold their newborns skin-to-skin are told to look for signs of hunger. They're told to watch for when baby starts turning his head, putting his hands to his mouth, licking his lips, yawning, and—if these early signs are missed—crying. But trying to interpret newborn gestures can be confusing. If you spend time, instead, relaxing in a reclined position with your newborn on your chest, you can just let baby latch and unlatch as he pleases.

Be intentional about "top-up" bottles.

A fed baby is more important than a breastfed baby.

Sometimes a bottle (of either formula or pumped breastmilk) is medically necessary. If doctors determine that your baby's weight gain and growth are not satisfactory, or if you have nipple damage or can't get baby to latch, then bottles may be required to help him thrive.[8]

But if your plan is to breastfeed and you haven't been told by a healthcare professional to provide a bottle for medical reasons, then you'll want to carefully consider whether bottles of formula or pumped milk are a good fit for your family right now.

Bottles make it harder to breastfeed.

A so-called "top-up" bottle never works as a supplement to your breastmilk. A bottle always functions, rather, as a *replacement* for your breastmilk. It's not a top-up bottle. It's an "instead-of" bottle.

And instead-of bottles have a tendency to undermine breastfeeding, especially in the early days.

To begin with, it's much easier to drink from a bottle than to drink from a breast. Milk essentially pours out of a bottle, whereas a baby has to engage in active suckling to get breastmilk from a breast. Almost every infant given both options will eventually reject the breast and pick the easier feeding method.

Secondly, a bottle nipple (regardless of the brand) isn't the same as a breast nipple. Baby needs one type of tongue action to empty a bottle

---

[8] If bottles are medically necessary but your plan had been to breastfeed, you can ask your health professionals for information and help. Some questions you could consider: Given that breastfed babies normally take in about 30 mL (one ounce) of colostrum during the first 24 hours of nursing, and not much more in the days immediately following the birth, how much formula is your baby going to get? What's the rationale for the amount being recommended? What variable will determine whether bottles are no longer necessary? If you reach a point where medical staff give you the green light to transition from bottles, can they recommend someone who can help you build (or rebuild) your milk production?

and another kind to empty a breast. If baby uses the tongue action that works on the bottle nipple on momma's breast, he'll push the breast out of his mouth and end up with a shallow latch, which could lead to painful nipple damage for mom and poor milk transfer for baby.

Finally, when baby is feeding from a bottle rather than suckling from a breast, momma's body doesn't get hormonal signals to make milk. And the effects are multiplied in an exponential feedback loop. A bottlefeeding tells your body to make less milk, but less breastmilk makes baby less interested in nursing, which sends your body the message to cut milk production further.

Breastfeeding is a supply-and-demand system: the more baby nurses (particularly in those crucial first 40 days when milk supply is being established), the more milk gets made.

Willingness to take a bottle doesn't imply hunger.

If you offer a bottle, a baby will *always* take it, even after a full feeding.

Remember, the tasty goodness you've put in the bottle (whether formula or pumped breastmilk) has been designed (by scientists or by nature) to be the ultimate, most delicious comfort food. It's sweet, it's creamy, and it makes baby feel so, so *goooooooood**. And since it's being offered in a bottle, your baby doesn't even have to work for it—it just flows right in!

Think of infant food (both formula and breastmilk) as a giant plate of nachos at a pub, or your favourite dessert at Thanksgiving. Regardless of how much you just ate, your brain sees that good stuff and makes the call: *Oh, surely I can squeeze in just a little bit more*!

Your baby is in the same boat: Heck, yeah, he'll find room for some cheese-slathered nachos!

Breastmilk in = Diapers out.

Over their first couple of days, newborn babies typically have one to two wet diapers and at least one or two poops. Your baby's first stools, called meconium, will be dark green—almost black. His first urine will be orange or rust-coloured and arrive in small amounts.

Somewhere between Day 3 and Day 5, once your milk has come in, baby's diaper output will increase to three or four wet diapers per day and at least three green, brown or yellow transitional poops per day. Soon after, your baby's urine should start arriving in larger amounts and take on a light yellow colour.

Swaddle your sweet baby, but only sometimes.

Swaddling has been around for thousands of years, and is practised around the world.

Swaddling involves tightly wrapping your baby in a large cloth or blanket.[9]

It's popular the world over because it works for calming a newborn. Newborn babies have a startle reflex, which can wake them from an otherwise peaceful sleep. Keeping your baby's arms bound in a swaddle can help prevent this reflex from waking him up.

Swaddling also reminds baby of the comforting confines of momma's womb, and keeps him warm, without the need for too many layers. In the first few weeks of life, many moms don't even bother dressing their babies under the swaddle. If you bundle your newborn in just a diaper and a swaddling blanket or two, then every time you pick up your little burrito for some babymoon time, all you need to do is unravel his blanket, and *voilà!* He's ready for bare-skin cuddling!

Swaddling isn't suited to all situations.

Swaddling is great, but there's a hitch. For mommas trying to build up their breastmilk supply, the **drawback** of swaddling is that **it works**. You read that right: The fact that swaddling works so well is a bit of a problem.

You see, babies who are swaddled sleep longer. While this might sound good, keep in mind that the more time your baby spends

---

[9] Here's a helpful video on how to swaddle: healthyparentshealthychildren.ca/resources/videos-injury-prevention-and-staying-healthy#swaddling.

sleeping in a contented swaddle, the less time he'll spend nursing. Which will make it that much harder for your milk supply to increase with his needs.

Plus, what are you going to do with your bundled baby while he lies in a bassinet all day? Just stare at him from afar?

Fortunately, this doesn't mean you should never swaddle your baby if you're a breastfeeding momma. After all, swaddling comes with one big **advantage**, which is that **it works**!

Just use it judiciously.

Experienced moms usually make generous use of the swaddle at nighttime. If health professionals have no concerns about your baby's growth (which means he's getting enough breastmilk), and he's sleeping on a separate surface,[10] then encouraging your baby to sleep longer at night sounds lovely. So at **nighttime**, consider confining your baby in a cozy swaddle.

But in the **daytime**, aim to spend less time like this…

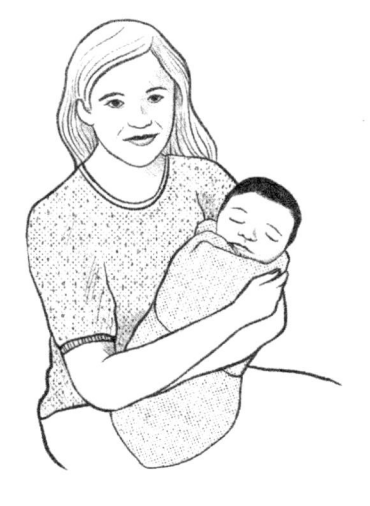

…and more time like this.

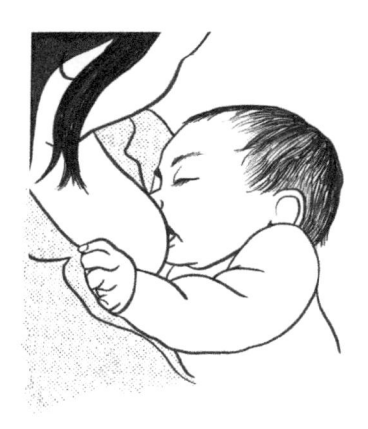

---

10   It's never safe to share a sleep surface with a swaddled baby. For the same reason, never breastfeed a swaddled baby at night. Instead, undo the swaddle and bring baby skin-to-skin before breastfeeding, just in case you fall asleep while nursing.

CHAPTER 5:
First Two Weeks

> "Sam has his mom—his universe—during that stage when 'attachment parenting' doesn't even begin to touch the glorious extremity of that new baby bond."
>
> –Nathan Englander, "We the North: On finding a home in Canada", *The Globe and Mail* (December 26, 2020)

You're still in the babymoon phase.

Remember when you were four and carried your dolls or stuffed animals around the house non-stop? Well, this is what you were practising for. This is it.

At this stage, both breastfeeding and sleeping continue to be baby-led. Everything's easier if momma simply follows baby's cues and offers to nurse him as much as he wants and soothes him to sleep as much as he needs. And the simplest way of making sure you never miss a feeding or sleeping cue is by continuing to spend as much time as possible reclined, with baby skin-to-skin and tummy-to-mommy.

You may be wondering around now how much longer this babymoon business is supposed to last. Answer: around 40 days. That's five and a half weeks. If you're reading this chapter before baby has arrived, take time now to book off the first 40 postpartum days on your calendar, the way you would a critical client meeting or a holiday.

Forty days can feel like forever, and many moms find it takes **about eight days** to let go and give in to the laidback rhythm of *il dolce far niente*—an Italian expression that roughly translates as "the sweetness of doing nothing."

It can be hard to step off the treadmill and give in to the sweetness of lounging around in bed all day. It's hard because when you've got lots of stuff to do—as we all do—you don't want to waste your time. But sitting back and embracing *il dolce far niente* in its many forms isn't wasteful. It's critical for establishing breastmilk supply.

It takes many hours of breastfeeding over the first 40 days after birth to establish full breastmilk supply. And it's impossible to breastfeed for hours and hours each day if you're running around getting other stuff done. So while lying around in bed with your baby may seem self-indulgent (best-case scenario) or slow, insular, and anxiety-inducing (worst-case scenario), remind yourself that you're not just lazing about—you're also breastfeeding.

Wake up—breakfast is ready!

Most moms begin to feel breast fullness and the sensation of milk coming in about three to five days after birth. To help alleviate fullness and discomfort in your breasts, try to feed your baby as much as possible once your milk comes in.

Many newborns also increase their awake and alert time around Day 3, 4, or 5, just as the milk comes in. After the darkness of momma's womb, babies mostly keep their eyes closed for the first few days after birth. But by Day 3, 4, or 5 they're getting used to the bright light. That's one explanation for the uptick in awake time. Another explanation, though, might be that your baby kept hitting the snooze button until breakfast was ready. Once your milk has come in, it's go time!

Dealing with engorgement (breasts that are *too* full of milk)

If your baby has trouble latching onto your fuller breasts, try expressing[11] a little milk—softer breasts are easier to latch on to.

In rare cases, moms experience painful engorgement around three to four days after birth. If your breasts become hard, heavy, hot, and swollen despite your best efforts to feed baby frequently, they may be engorged.

Moms are at greatest risk for engorgement if they used a breast pump over the first few days. If your baby is nursing *and* you're pumping, then you're effectively telling your body to make lots and lots of milk. Too much milk. More milk than your baby can consume or your body can handle.

If you experience engorgement, avoid using a breast pump for relief unless advised to do so by a health professional—it could make the problem worse. In the meantime, here are some suggestions for alleviating painful engorgement without a pump:

- Spend time in bed, skin-to-skin, and encourage your baby to nurse as much as possible.

- Hand express milk in the shower. If you're quite engorged, your breasts will likely start dripping into the hot water without your help. You can also massage your breasts gently, concentrating on any lumps or sore areas, and directing a circular motion from armpit to nipple.

- Fill a large bowl with hot water (as in hot-tub hot), lean forward over the bowl with your breast submerged, and hand express into the bowl.[12]

---

11   Here's an excellent video, if you need a visual: med.stanford.edu/newborns/professional-education/breastfeeding/hand-expressing-milk.html

12   If you're hand expressing in the shower or into a towel or bowl of warm water, you may wonder if it isn't more prudent to express this precious milk into containers for freezing. Short answer: it isn't. Many a first-time mom has ended up tossing out the litres of unused frozen breastmilk at the back of her freezer. For now, just focus on establishing your breastmilk supply and getting to know your baby. Collecting breastmilk for those times when you're apart from baby is very easy and not something you need to worry about now.

- Place a cold compress on your breast to reduce swelling and relieve pain. Protect your skin by wrapping an ice pack, gel pack, or bag of frozen vegetables in a cloth and applying it to your breasts for about 20 minutes or so. A cold compress is more for pain relief than anything else—on its own it won't resolve the engorgement.

- Clean, dry, and chill several cabbage leaves, then place pieces of them in your bra. Cover the entire surface of the affected breast, but not your nipple, for about 20 minutes or so, and then discard.

- Take a mild pain medication such as acetaminophen (less than 1 percent of which gets passed on to your baby).

- While breastfeeding, massage your breasts to help the milk flow. Gently massage any lumpy areas.

- If a lump has formed in your breast due to a blocked milk duct, change baby's position so that his chin is between your nipple and the lump. Your baby drains milk most efficiently from the area around his chin because of the strong sucking motion of his lower jaw.

Blocked ducts that go undrained and persistent engorgement can put you at risk of *mastitis*—an inflammation of the breast that can progress to an infection with flu-like symptoms. While mastitis usually clears up quickly with treatment by a medical professional, you'll make your life easier if you deal with any blocked ducts and engorgement as soon as they appear, before mastitis has a chance to develop. Prevention is worth a pound of cure!

If the engorgement persists, seek help.

Most breastfeeding challenges can be solved with information and support, so if breastfeeding doesn't feel good in any way, it's best to get help quickly. For suggested helpers, see the Resources section near the end of this book, or the chapter on breastfeeding.

After your milk comes in, breastfeeding will ease back from taking up eight hours per 24-hour day.

As your milk production and the size of your baby's stomach both steadily grow, by Day 3 or 4 you might find that breastfeeding is beginning to take up slightly less of your day. Your baby's feedings may also be getting somewhat shorter by the end of the first week, and he may be satisfied for longer stretches. This is something that happens on its own. Momma doesn't need to do anything different to make the feedings shorter or to space them out. Your newborn knows his own needs and abilities and will take the lead on breastfeeding frequency and duration.

But even though it no longer takes up eight hours per day, nursing continues to be frequent and unpredictable.

By Week 2, your baby's stomach capacity will increase to the size of a large chicken egg, and this rapid growth will continue for a few more weeks.

The most effective way to increase your milk supply in tandem with your baby's growing appetite is to sit around and nurse. Nothing works as well as a baby at the breast for increasing milk supply. Not Domperidone. Not breast pumps. Not special tea. Not Guinness. Just good old-fashioned skin-to-skin time at the breast.

The more frequently a baby nurses in the first few weeks, the more prolactin receptors develop in the glandular cells of the breast, and the more milk momma will make. As an added protective bonus, the more prolactin receptors you lay down in the first few weeks, the more easily your breastmilk supply will adjust to future fluctuations in your baby's feeding demands. In other words, the more time you dedicate to breastfeeding now, the easier breastfeeding will be later.

If you're getting help from someone who's not familiar with breastfeeding, they may give you incorrect advice that you should try to schedule your baby's feedings. But a momma breastfeeding a newborn baby can no more schedule a feeding than she can schedule a diaper change. Feedings and diaper changes are crazy frequent at this stage, but this will not be your new normal. The pace and frequency of feedings and diaper changes will eventually decrease on their own, just not yet. You're more likely to reach your breastfeeding goals if you go along with your newborn's inefficient feeding pattern and let him figure out a more predictable nursing schedule on his own. He's working on it, Momma! He'll get there!

Suck-suck-suck-suck-suck-suck-paaaaaause

Babies' suckling tends to follow a pattern. They suck, swallow, suck, swallow, suck, swallow, suck, swallow… and then pause. The pause doesn't mean they're done. Wait a bit… And the pattern will likely start all over again.

Toddlers using soothers follow this same sequence (but without the "swallow" bit). Even *The Simpsons*' observant animators took care to give Maggie the same suck-suck-suck-suck-pause pattern with her ever-present soother!

Each batch of milk you produce is artisanal.

Your breastmilk will continue changing as your baby grows, because your body custom-produces artisanal batches for every feed, adjusting aspects such as fat content and antibodies as needed.

One change you may notice around Week 2 is in the colour of your milk; it will start looking a lot thinner and more blue than the milk you were making last week. Bluish milk is perfectly normal at this stage. Human milk looks different from cow milk!

Weight gain in baby is the most reliable indicator of whether momma is making enough milk.

Moms are more likely to meet their breastfeeding goals if they're aware that weight gain is the only reliable indicator of whether baby is getting enough breastmilk to feel satisfied and full.

As I mentioned in the previous chapter, it is normal for your baby to lose weight in the first three to five days after birth, before your milk comes in. Your baby's lowest weight will likely occur between

Day 3 and Day 5. After that there should be a gradual increase every day. Most babies gain between 20 and 35 g (2/3 and 1¼ oz) per day between Day 6 and Day 13. Even with this steady increase, though, by the end of Week 1 your baby's weight could still be lower than his birth weight.

Most breastfed babies regain their birth weight between Days 10 and 14. If yours hasn't regained his birth weight by Day 14, that's a red flag, and you should ask a medical professional for help.

On the other hand, **if your baby *has* regained his birth weight *by Day 14*, and health professionals are satisfied with his overall growth, then you can rest assured he's getting enough breastmilk.** You're doing it!

> ### Good to know!
>
> Expect 24- to 48-hr intense feeding when baby has growth spurts at one, three, and six weeks & at three months.
>
> During his growth spurts, you'll notice that your baby wants to nurse much more often. Sometimes it will feel like all day long! This is normal and expected.
>
> After two or three days, your baby should return to his previous pattern of breastfeeding and seem more content.

There's no such thing as a wasted feeding.

Any and all nursing at this stage will help increase your milk supply and help your baby grow.

But it's not just about milk volume and weight gain. Another benefit of frequent breastfeeding is that it makes your baby feel good. As adults, food isn't purely about calories. It's about sharing, celebrating, and connecting. It's one of life's great pleasures! Nursing, similarly, is your baby's first experience with food as a social connection.

If you try to treat nursing as a social connection, too, it might help you find the Zen of this time together: The lightweight beauty of your baby, the repetitiveness of the feeding motions, the satisfaction of a fed baby, and the peacefulness of curling up in your comforter while the many items on your usual to-do list fall away for several weeks.

Lots of breastmilk in = lots of filled diapers out.

Between Day 3 and Day 5, your baby will probably produce three to four really wet diapers and at least three green, brown or yellow transitional poops in each 24-hour period.

After about Day 6, most breastfed newborns produce six or more heavy, wet diapers per day and at least three large, soft and seedy poops.

Seedy?

Yes, seedy. It's normal for breastfed babies to have watery, yellow, seedy stool. Green, spinach-like stool isn't uncommon either.

You'll also be dealing with poopy diapers in the middle of the night. When they're a few days old, newborns start pooping *a lot*, including during the night. Expect to do several nighttime diaper changes during the first few weeks, but rest assured that this will not be your new normal. As your baby grows and develops, he'll naturally develop the ability to "hold it in" for increasing periods and eliminate less often. And in a few weeks your baby will achieve his *first* milestone on the way to full toilet-training—the ability to control his bowels at night. When that happy day arrives, you'll no longer have to change poopy diapers at night.

While you're waiting for him to hit these various milestones, changing diapers often will keep your baby comfortable and help prevent diaper rash. All in, between the nighttime and daytime nappy changes, you're probably looking at close to a dozen diapers daily at the newborn stage.

Give baby a quick clean when needed, which won't be often.

A bath or shower once per week or so is likely more than enough until your child hits the pre-teen years (or starts playing hockey!).

And when you soap your baby, focus on the bits that actually need it, because there's no rule that says the entire body needs to be lathered during a bath or shower.

In her book *Beyond Soap*, dermatologist Dr. Sandy Skotnicki makes the case for minimizing (not avoiding—just minimizing) the use of soaps, cleansers, and balms in order to give skin a fighting chance to maintain the baseline state that biology intended. Each of hosts an estimated 100 trillion micro-organisms on and in our bodies. We're not just individuals; we're ecosystems. According to Dr. Skotnicki, daily rinsing with hot water and soap can strip away lipids, alter our skin's microbiome, and potentially increase reactions to irritants and allergens.

As recently as the 1940s, eczema—inflamed, scaly, itchy skin—was relatively rare, affecting just 5 percent of children and comparatively unknown in adults. Today, higher proportions of young people and adults suffer from this condition. Damage to the skin's barrier function has also been associated with an increasing incidence of asthma, hay fever, and food hypersensitivities, including peanut allergies. To be clear, association is not the same as causation. No one knows what causes allergies, eczema, and weird, persistent rashes. It's possible, though, that frequent soaping could be a contributing factor.

Most children won't experience skin problems from a daily bath, but among the small minority of children with a genetic predisposition to eczema, asthma, or allergies, a daily bath could be a contributing factor to developing a reaction. We don't know who'll be susceptible, so why take the risk? Frequent washing can be hard on a baby's sensitive skin.

Try putting your baby in a baby carrier.

The first couple of weeks are a good time to try putting your baby in a carrier. Many moms find it easier to figure out how to use one in the privacy of their own home, before going out in public.

If you haven't considered getting a baby carrier, let me give you a bit of a pitch. Baby carriers can make your life easier in lots of ways, from soothing to burping to getting from Point A to Point B.

Transportation

As a means of getting around, a quality baby carrier has several advantages over a stroller:

- ✓ You'll be able to weave through crowds more nimbly.

- ✓ You'll be able to go up and down stairs easily. Heavy snow won't slow you down either. With a stroller, you're basically restricted to wheelchair-accessible parts of your environment.

- ✓ It's faster to toss a baby carrier onto the front seat of your car than to fold down a collapsible stroller and wedge it into your trunk.

Part of the beauty of a quality baby carrier is the years of use you'll get out of it. Though you'll use it far less frequently once baby begins to walk, it'll still be useful for the odd long-distance haul well into his third year. It's easier to set off on, say, a hike in the mountains if you know your two-year-old can be placed in the carrier once he's tuckered out.

And it should go without saying that a child is never too old for the carrier. They'll be too big one day, yes, but that's about physical size. As long as they fit in the carrier, they're exactly the right age for it.

Of course, this isn't a knock against strollers, which are also fabulous as transportation devices. I'm simply saying that adding a carrier to your mobility repertoire can expand your options.

Soothing

Carriers are great for transportation, but they have an even more important use—they calm your baby. It may seem counter-intuitive, but many parents use a baby carrier to soothe their baby *inside* their home more often than they use it *outside* their home for transportation. Newborns are blessedly content in the snug hold of a carrier on your chest, and fretful toddlers can often be calmed when strapped to your back.

Carriers work as soothing devices because human infants thrive on touch, motion, and closeness with their caregivers. When heard up close, the rhythm of an adult's heartbeat gives your baby calming neurological cues. He's also wired to find the vibrations and predictable, serve-and-return cadence of your inhalations, exhalations, and conversations calming—particularly, again, when heard up close.

So even if you prefer to use a stroller when you're out and about, consider getting a baby carrier for when you're at home, as a baby-pacifying device.

Reducing pressure on a newborn's soft skull

When your newborn is in a carrier, he's not lying down and putting pressure on the back of his head, the way he would be in a bucket seat, bouncy seat, or pram. This means that all the time your baby spends in his carrier counts towards the daily "tummy time" that health professionals recommend so that newborns won't develop flat areas on their heads.

Burping

Instead of having you sit around and pat his back for a burping, your baby can work out any air he's swallowed by spending time in a carrier. Babies tend to be less fussy when they're upright after a feeding.

Napping

During baby's first four months, many moms use the carrier as a mobile daytime napping device so they can get out of the house and explore the neighbourhood with their snoozy woozy newborn.

So, why is this a good time to try out the baby carrier?

Around the 14-days-old mark, there's a very good chance your baby will begin crying uncontrollably for no good reason (fun times!). When this happens, walking around your house with baby in the carrier is one of the tools you can reach for, so it's a good idea to practise putting him in it now (during the first two weeks, while he's still a "good baby"), instead of waiting until next week—when all hell is going to break loose.

But for now, during the first two weeks, it's usually fairly simple to soothe a newborn.

During your baby's first two weeks of life, he should never have **unsoothable** crying. "Unsoothable crying" means crying that parents can't soothe away, no matter what they try.

If your baby cries, try picking him up.

If that doesn't work, offer to nurse.

If that doesn't work, see if baby wants a *thicker* blanket or a *lighter* blanket over his back as he snuggles in skin-to-skin with you or dad.

If that doesn't work, try changing baby's diaper.

If that doesn't work, try putting baby down and swaddling him for warmth and coziness.

If you cannot soothe baby, then ask a medical professional for help.

Caring for a newborn can seem complicated at times, but in many ways it's quite simple. Barring a medical issue, when baby is <u>less than two weeks old</u> you should be able to soothe away all tears using the suggestions above, which can be further simplified to the following four actions:

1. Nursing to address his hunger or his need to be soothed into sleep.

2. Changing his dirty diaper to address his discomfort.

3. Picking him up and holding him skin-to-skin or in a baby carrier or simply in your arms, to address his need for security.

4. Putting him down, possibly in a swaddle, to address his need for deep sleep.

That's it. That's all you need. That, and some confidence that ***you*** are fully qualified to take care of all of your baby's needs with just these four solutions.

What you don't need is colic medicine, home-made remedies, homeopathic tinctures, robotic bassinets, smartphone-enabled shushing sounds, or chiropractic spinal manipulation. You don't need to second-guess your own diet, or how you're positioning baby for nursing or what side you place baby on when you put him down. You don't need to track the start and end of every feed and snooze on an app.

You can do it, Momma, without any magic potions and lotions.

Let your baby sleep like a baby.

A frequent and unpredictable sleeping pattern is still expected.

During the first couple of weeks, there's no discernable pattern to a baby's day- or nighttime sleep. It doesn't matter if your baby just woke up from a five-minute or a five-hour slumber—there's no way of knowing whether his next snooze will be in two minutes or in two hours.

It's also not possible to sleep-train at this stage.

It *will* be possible to sleep-train baby when he's a bit older—just not yet.

Help your baby figure out day and night.

While it's too early for sleep-training, it's not too early for parents to gradually set the stage for sleep-training later on.

Daytime naps are a good place to start. Your baby isn't clear on the difference between night sleep and day sleep yet, but you are. Since your ultimate goal is to get baby on board with regular, big-people sleep/wake rhythms, let's begin by referring to his daytime sleeps as "naps."

See—you're not trying to impose anything on baby yet. You're simply adjusting your vocabulary. We're going to do this whole sleep thing in baby steps, Momma!

It's also not a bad idea to keep his surroundings dark at night (even when he's awake) but let your baby hang out in well-lit conditions during the daytime (even when he's asleep). Things will work out better *later on* if your baby has a dark environment for his daytime naps, but at **the newborn stage** a bright-all-day environment is best during the daylight hours.

The circadian rhythm is the 24-hour cycle that keeps our body's functions running on time, including the secretion of melatonin to promote sleep. The human circadian rhythm isn't fully developed at birth, but the right environmental stimulus will help kick it into gear. When light hits the retina in our eyes, it signals the brain that it's day and not night. To get your newborn baby on board with normal circadian rhythms, minimize bright lights at night and avoid drawn shades in the daytime for the first three or four months.

Watch for signs of sleep readiness.

Nurse your baby to sleep whenever you observe signs of sleepiness, which can include eye rubbing, yawning, head turning, and crankiness. You may also notice his arm and leg movements slow down, his eyes become less sparkly, and that he seems less interested in you. A newborn will **usually** show signs of drowsiness after **one to two hours** of wakefulness (although it's also normal for a newborn to have both shorter and longer stretches of wakefulness).

Potential daytime-nap locations

When your newborn falls asleep in the daytime, you have three nap locations to choose from:

- **Babymoon nap.** Baby can sleep in your arms, since you may be spending many hours in bed together.
- **Baby-carrier nap.** You can let your baby nap in a carrier.
- **Bassinet or blankie nap.** You can put your baby down for a nap on any safe sleep surface.

Any of these three options is fine. None will create long-term habits at this stage.

And none of these three options is more "natural" or "better." While you're still in the babymoon phase during the first week, many moms start to get restless by this point and want to spend more of their daytime hours up and about. This is a perfectly normal progression.

Just pick whatever option *you* prefer in the moment, Momma.

You can even change your mind midway through the nap and pick up baby and stick him in a baby carrier, or put him down in a bassinet.[13] At this age, the transfer from one sleep surface to another is unlikely to wake your baby.

Make some noise.

Whatever location you choose for daytime naps, make sure you keep the house busy and full of regular daytime sounds. Go in and out of the room he's sleeping in. Leave his door open. Set up a sleep spot for him in the living room if you like. Don't fuss about guests who ring the doorbell. Invite a friend over for coffee. Tune in to talk radio or a podcast. Don't shush your loud-talking sister when she comes to admire her brand-new niece or nephew.

During their first three or four months, babies sleep more soundly when they can hear the regular din of their kinfolk around them.

Newborn babies go to bed very late in the evening.

Kind of too late, really, for a momma who's now officially short on sleep.

Once baby goes to sleep for the night, starting sometime between 9 pm and midnight at this stage, turn off the lights and turn down the noise. Now momma can finally go to bed!

During the first couple of weeks, you can expect your baby to wake up frequently throughout the night to breastfeed. You'll want to keep the lights dim (or use a flashlight or nightlight) for these night feedings.

---

13 By *bassinet*, I'm referring to any safe sleep surface set up in mom and dad's bedroom that's separate from mom and dad's bed. It could be a portable Pack n' Play,™ a side-sleeper that attaches to your adult mattress, a crib, an actual bassinet, or a sturdy box. It doesn't matter. The key is that it's a separate sleep surface, just for baby.

Your baby still isn't clear on this whole day/night thing, but he'll slowly get the picture that, at night, it's dark and eerily quiet, the world is mind-numbingly dull, and momma takes just a wee bit longer to respond when he stirs.

Check on your soundly sleeping baby! What's that strange snorting sound?!

Many newborn babies make weird gargling, gurgling goat noises when they sleep.

If it's getting to be too much, you can pick him up and hold him for a while. This may help regulate his breathing. Your other option is to just quickly check on baby, reassure yourself he's all right, and go back to bed.

By and large, newborns' weird grunting goat noises are normal and expected. But they're very, very unnerving.

"But wait!," you say, "How will I know the difference between a gargling, gurgling sound that signifies serious medical distress and a gargling, gurgling sound that's as normal and expected as the borborygmi of a rumbling stomach? What's the difference? When should I get worried?"

I don't have the answer to that. (But hey, that was a sweet use of *borborygmi* in a sentence.)

The reality is—now that you've had a baby—that perpetual, low-grade anxiety spiked with occasional outright panic you've been feeling isn't going to end any time soon. It's not just the nocturnal goat noises that you'll worry over. It's everything. Is this rash a problem? Will that lunatic driver fail to stop in time? Rusty nails? Tick invasions? *Respiratory syncytial virus?!*

If you're worried, you can always ask a medical professional to check your baby.

Otherwise, take a deep breath in, blow it out, and use your newborn's gargling goat noises to practise the art of constantly reassuring yourself that everything is fine.

Everything is fine.

Everything is definitely (maybe) fine.

Sleep in.

In these initial weeks, some moms manage to "sleep in" after the early morning feeds. Perhaps you'll be able to as well.

If you can stay in bed from, say, midnight to 10 am, then even with frequent night feedings you might be able to sneak in seven hours of shut-eye during this 10-hour period and make up for some of that lost, precious middle-of-the-night sleep.

In the mornings, newborns tend to cycle between sleeping and calm, alert time. In other words, they rarely cry at this time of day. This means the early morning can be a lovely time for grandma and grandpa to come over and enjoy some one-on-one bonding with their new grandchild, while you finish loading up on the sleep hours you were denied last night.

Notice that baby is still here. Surreal.

During their first few days of motherhood, many moms enter a fugue state that combines both high alertness and meditative languor.

Removed from the rhythms of your normal routine
You may find that you're fully
Aware
Of
Each
Moment
While the hours slip by
In a liminal
Fog

Be forewarned that this intensely charged but dreamlike postnatal period isn't always a good thing. A millstone of free-floating dread can sometimes envelop a new mom.

The term "overview effect" is used in space exploration to describe the cognitive shift that can happen when astronauts view our planet from outer space and feel struck by the fragility of the thin blue line that makes possible all life on Earth. For many space explorers, the overview effect brings home the insignificance of our human preoccupations.

A mother cradling her newborn baby can experience a similar transcendental overview effect. It's not uncommon for a new mom to become suddenly aware of—and then to feel awed, or even overwhelmed by—the thin line separating the miracle from the tragedy of human life.

In our normal day-to-day we can push these thoughts out of our minds, but birth is a stark reminder of our mortality. When you've just witnessed someone being born it's hard to gloss over the reality that we're also all going to die.

This is the abyss, and you've glimpsed it: When two people embrace the deepest form of love, it will *always* end with grief.

> You and your baby will not always be okay.
>
> One of you will go first.
>
> And whoever is left will be devastated.

In the days following birth, your primitive, mammalian self can become alert to the fragility (and futility) of *everything*.

Instead of fighting against this rising tide of existential angst, let it wash over you, and then regroup. You're okay. You've got this.

For most moms, this period of magnified perceptivity will pass on its own and you'll soon go back to sweating the small stuff. If it doesn't pass and you suspect you've caught a case of postpartum depression, seek help from a medical professional.

Postpartum depression has a profound effect on the entire family, but it's a treatable medical condition. One translation of that quote from Friedrich Nietzsche, "If you gaze long into the abyss, the abyss gazes back into you,"[14] is this: Don't stare into the void for too long. Get help from a doctor before it swallows you up.

---

14   Source: *Beyond Good and Evil,* 1886, by Friedrich Nietzsche (1844-1900)

CHAPTER 6:

Day 14 to Day 40

> "'Well, what is it for?' said the man. 'It is for loving and hugging and feeding and burping', said Robin."
>
> —by Robert Munsch, excerpt from his classic picture book, *Murmel, Murmel, Murmel* (1982)

Don't just do something. Sit there...

...And breastfeed.

The babymoon period lasts 40 days, so you're in the homestretch now. For these next three weeks, continue to spend as much time as possible reclined, with baby skin-to-skin and tummy-to-mommy.

Your body is still increasing the amount of breastmilk it produces—but the finish line is in sight.

During the first 40 days of your baby's life, two things happen: each day, you make more breastmilk than the previous day, and each day, baby's capacity to consume that breastmilk increases.

By about Day 40, in the normal course of breastfeeding, mothers hit their peak milk production. After that, your breastmilk supply will stay more or less the same. That's because from about the age of one month to about the age of six months, your baby will need approximately the same amount of breastmilk every day. After about Day 40, your breastmilk production can still increase slightly if, say, your baby nurses more often during a growth spurt, during a heat wave, or while fighting a cold. In general, though, the volume of milk you produce should be pretty steady after Day 40.

> **Good to know!**
>
> Expect 24 to 48 hours of increased feeding when baby has growth spurts at one, three, six weeks & at three months.

So keep in mind how important these first 40 days are for establishing breastmilk production. If your goal is to nurse your baby exclusively for about the first five or six months, then it helps to keep at it for the first five or six weeks and to nurse as often as possible.

Weight gain is still the most reliable indicator of whether your baby is getting enough breastmilk.

If health professionals are satisfied with your baby's weight gain and growth then you can rest assured that your baby is getting enough breastmilk.

Poopy diapers are a secondary, less reliable indicator. If, in his first four weeks, your breastfed baby is having fewer than four stools a day *and* those stools are firm, you should make an appointment with your doctor, who can check whether baby is feeding well and whether there are problems with his bowel. Between Day 14 and Day 40, breastfed newborns typically have at least three large, soft and seedy yellow poops—and at least six heavy, wet diapers.

Empty breasts make more milk.

Breastmilk is produced almost continuously. In the mid-20th century, moms were sometimes erroneously advised to wait and give their breasts a chance to "fill up." But our breasts aren't like milk bottles that get drained. Your body is ready to produce more milk even if you just finished nursing and it feels like baby got every last drop.

Empty breasts tell your body to make more milk. Pronto!

Full breasts tell your body to *sloooow doooown* milk production.

Instead of looking for hunger signs, pretend your baby is a guest at a fabulous party you're hosting.

When you're the host of a gathering, you don't look for hunger signs in your guests. Instead, you just keep offering: "Have some more salad. Would you like another beer? How about I top up your glass? I'm just going to slide this bowl of chips towards you." That's the mindset you need at this stage. Keep offering.

A babymoon is good for a momma's post-birthing recovery.

Remember that taking a babymoon for the first 40 days after birth doesn't just help build breastmilk supply. It also helps your body rest up and physically recover from childbirth. If one month postpartum you still look *pregnant*, it's a sign the rest of you isn't back to normal yet either. So even though you *can* get up and vacuum the whole house, you *shouldn't*. Ease up on things.

A babymoon helps minimize a visitor free-for-all.

Another benefit of a babymoon is that it helps remind everyone that baby's first six weeks are a private time for him and momma. Visitors should expect that, if they pop by, you and your baby may be squirrelled away napping in your bedroom, your baby nearly naked and

> **Good to know!**
>
> Mommas have a vaginal discharge called lochia that lasts for up to six weeks after the birth of a baby. Lochia is caused by the uterus shedding and renewing its lining. For the first two to five days, the flow will be red. By five to 10 days, the flow will usually turn pink, then brown. After 10 days, the flow is generally either white or colourless.
>
> You may need to stock up on heavier pads than you normally use.
>
> To help prevent infection, avoid using tampons for the first six weeks after birth.

you dishevelled. The babymoon tucks you away in a cozy mum-and-bub bubble.

The payoff

If you can make it through these first 40 days, you'll end up with an easy-peasy, well-established breastfeeding relationship with your baby. It may be an intense time-investment now, but once the 40 days are up, you're done! The babymoon phase will be over.

A babymoon helps re-set a mom's expectations.

The seeming lack of accomplishment during this enforced relaxation period helps reset a mom's expectations for how much can get done in a day. Before baby arrived, you might have thought a year-long maternity leave would provide an excellent opportunity to efficiently work through your to-do list. After all, you're a woman of ambition. You know how to multitask.

But the reality is that, for the first year or so, even once your babymoon is done, you'll probably only have time for one non-baby-related task per day. Just one. Make dinner. Or catch up on social media. Or mop. Or switch out the winter tires. Or visit with friends. Pick one.

This can feel frustrating for a working woman accustomed to producing more, at a far faster pace, while on the job. Many moms engaged in the mundane minutiae of babycare get the nagging feeling that they should be working on something else. Idleness doesn't feel right, because we're conditioned to always doing, doing, doing.

"Being" is a whole lot harder than "doing." And the reality is that *being* mom is your new full-time job.

And it's a full-time job with no satisfying list of accomplishments to check off to gauge progress. Every diaper change, every breastfeeding, every sleep-soothing, every grocery-store visit, every meal prep, every high-chair wiping carries no weight, because it's immediately replaced on the to-do list by the next diaper change, breastfeeding, sleep-soothing, grocery list, meal prep, and high-chair wiping. And in this never-ending loop of minutiae there's next to no time to spare.

It's a full-time job where all the tasks seem disjointed, and there's no sense of completion. Your old Monday-to-Friday gig with delineated start times, end times, and milestones has morphed into an endless, undefined mass.

Even calling new motherhood a full-time "job" isn't quite accurate. It's not a job. It's not an activity. You don't *do* motherhood. This explains why you feel like you're not getting anything *done*.

Taking a babymoon for the first 40 days or so after birth can feel overwhelming because we're conditioned to believe that productive adults wouldn't spend a month just lying around in bed.

But the conspicuous idleness of a babymoon can also help you recalibrate. You've brought a little person into your world. Everything, absolutely *everything*, has changed. Even if this is your second or third child, there's still value in slowing down to focus on this brand-new addition.

And it's not like a babymoon is devoid of concrete milestones. Look at what you're getting done: You're growing a human being! A human being well on his way to *doubling* his birth weight by the age of five months, and then tripling it by his first birthday!

It may seem ironic, but doing nothing takes some doing. It requires planning, and some new habits. You'll need to clear space in your calendar to make this babymoon possible. It's up to you to make it happen.

A babymoon can help slow a busy momma down and reset her expectations about what can be knocked off in a day. Your new daily to-do list should realistically have just two items on it each day:

✓ Parent your baby

✓ Pick one other thing.

Keep putting baby down for daytime naps.

As with breastfeeding, your baby's sleep continues to have no predictable pattern at this stage. There's no set daytime schedule. There's no set nighttime schedule. Just go with the flow.

In terms of timing, put your baby down whenever you observe signs of drowsiness. If he's getting a glassy look to his eyes, turning his head, batting at his face, slowing his movements, or starting to fuss, it may be time to nurse him back to sleep. Most of the time, babies at this age show sleepy signs after one to two hours of wakefulness, but the wakefulness span can also be much shorter or much longer. You'll want to watch your baby more than the clock.

For **daytime naps**, you can continue to let baby sleep in your arms, or put baby down on a separate sleep surface, or let baby nap in a carrier. None of these approaches will create long-term habits, and none is better or worse than another. Go with what feels right in the moment.

And pack away the baby monitor for now. People use monitors to amplify their baby's sounds. But that's also the problem with baby monitors: they amplify the baby's sounds, so you'll be rushing into his room at every gurgle and squeak. Do yourself—and baby—a big favour and unplug it. Trust me, if baby actually needs you, you *will* hear him.

Keep putting baby down for nighttime sleeps.

As with the previous week, when baby falls asleep for the night, turn off the lights and turn down the noise.

There's still no predictable pattern to night-waking and night-nursing at this stage. Your baby is still at an age when you need to nurse on demand, both day and night. Because newborns need to feed every few hours, you can expect approximately three night wakings—or more—over the course of each night. Expect repeated night-wakings, but don't expect them to form any consistent pattern.

There is one aspect of night-sleep, though, that does become fairly predictable between the ages of two weeks and 40 days: **your baby may start to stick to a fairly regular bedtime.** This bedtime will likely take place relatively late, somewhere between 9 pm and midnight. And it's a bedtime that baby picks—not you.

If you're lucky, your baby may be happy just hanging out with you and your partner while you watch TV in the evening.[15] If that's the case, then at least your baby isn't being much of a bother when he's up late.

If you're not lucky, then sometime after the age of two weeks your baby will turn into a holy terror in the evening hours. More on that later…

Go ahead and nurse your baby to sleep.

Right about now, someone may give you some well-meaning advice to "never nurse your baby to sleep." In other words, they may tell you to "always put your baby down drowsy but awake."

This isn't just bad advice, it's unfounded.

Some people falsely assume that nursing their baby to sleep will impede night-weaning or sleep-training later on. It won't. Nursing your baby to sleep at this stage will have no impact whatsoever on his future ability to sleep through the night.

Here's the analogy you can give to people who tell you otherwise: Like most adults, you probably have a soothing, nighttime ritual before you go to sleep at night. Maybe you watch TV. Maybe you read a book for twenty minutes. Whatever it is, it's probably hard for you to imagine falling asleep without it. Then, throughout the night, your mind arouses several times as you go through normal nighttime sleep cycles. You might hardly notice these arousals, which we all experience, because you've figured out how to get back to sleep without

---

15 This doesn't count as screen time for baby, because your newborn will be watching you and not the television.

your bedtime ritual. In other words, you don't need to get up to read or watch TV in the middle of the night to fall back into slumber.

The same applies to your baby. When he's ready to night-wean (not yet!), he'll be able to distinguish between the *beginning*-of-the-night-soothing-to-sleep routine (breastfeeding) versus whatever he'll draws on in the *middle* of the night to go back to sleep (which will be his job to figure out—not yours).

So, nursing your baby to sleep has no downsides.

And guess what—it gets better! Not only are there no downsides—there's one huge upside.

The advantage of nursing your baby to sleep is that it's fast and easy.

Parents who don't breastfeed their babies to sleep have to come up with other rituals—bathe baby, rock baby, sing to baby, play a smart-phone-connected music-box gizmo for baby, jiggle baby. Stroller rides, car rides, lavender oils, lullaby apps. Judging from the number of baby-soothing products available out there, soothing a baby to sleep without breastfeeding can be pretty labour-intensive.

Nursing your baby to sleep is one of your new momma super-powers. Go ahead and use it!

Start taking your own sweet time getting up at night.

Ok, so we're all on the same page. Breastfeeding needs to be "on demand" at this stage. When baby wakes up at night and cries, you need to nurse.

But you know what else is "on demand"? Momma's need to sleep.

And right about now the tender joy of a new baby is starting to wear thin in the middle of the night.

Which is fine. It's your body's way of saying, "Yeah, yeah, yeah, I'm still going to nurse baby. But in a minute. Just give me another minute."

Picture a cantankerous old man. How would *he* respond to this crying-baby-in-the-middle-of-the-night? That's right, Momma: you need to channel a bit of cranky old man.

It's a delicate balance.

Don't make your baby wait unnecessarily long for a nighttime feeding. You're not trying to teach him a lesson.

But <u>after about the first two weeks</u>, as long as health professionals are satisfied with your baby's weight gain and growth, it's okay if you sometimes don't *immediately* jump to attention in the middle of the night.

If you indiscriminately jump up to nurse every single time your baby calls out, you run the risk of misinterpreting nighttime murmurs and dream talk as hunger cries, and inadvertently fragmenting your child's sleep.

Maybe, sometimes, just give it a minute.

At night, do a good enough job. Then move on.

On a somewhat related note, during these first 40 days your baby may undergo a bit of a behavioural shift in the middle of the vast, dark night. Until now he's been happy to nurse back to sleep every time. But one night soon you might find yourself with a baby who won't go down after breastfeeding. You offer him one breast and he nurses and nurses.

Still awake.

So then you offer him the other breast and nurse him for what seems like the usual amount of time for a nighttime nursing. And then…

He's still awake!

Undeterred, you put him in his bassinet. Surely he'll fall asleep soon. After all, you've done what has worked every night until now. You've done a good enough job. You've given him his soothing milkie. The lights are all out. It's clearly night time. So you get back in your bed and try to go back to sleep.

And then he starts to cry.

So, you pick him up. Maybe try nursing again, but for a shorter time.

Put him down again. He's still awake. He cries again.

This is the point at which many families that hadn't planned on co-sleeping inadvertently slip into it.[16] And it's true: if you bring your baby into bed with you at this point, he'll stop crying. But if sharing a sleep surface isn't your plan, then you need to be aware that this is a normal and expected development and that you can power through it. This crying-every-time-you-put-him-down isn't going to be the new normal. You just need to get over the hump.

If you prefer to keep using separate sleep surfaces, reassure yourself, first, that you've done a really good job breastfeeding your baby—you've done what you can! You've clearly responded to his need for a middle-of-the-night nursing (and maybe a diaper change).

After giving yourself this little pep talk, try the following three fixes.

Fix #1: Allow your baby to express his strongly held preference for a co-sleeping family.

Put him back in his bassinet, where he is safe, and leave him there, even though he's crying. Go back to your bed and lie down. See if you can sleep. (Amazingly, even when baby is crying, many moms can get a few minutes of shut-eye in this type of situation if they're exhausted enough.)

If you find it hard to put your baby down, keep in mind that **you're not going to leave him crying for too long**. It's too early to sleep-train. You just need a bit of space. You've done your best, you've already tried breastfeeding him to sleep a few times, you're very, very tired, and you just need a little time to regroup.

---

16 Families have practised bed-sharing for millennia. If your plan is to share a bed, then go ahead and share a bed. I'm talking here about the families who inadvertently fall into bed-sharing when baby is a few weeks old even though they weren't planning on it, and then struggle to get baby out. The information in this section is intended for families who prefer to maintain separate sleep surfaces.

Fix #2: Try to soothe baby without nursing.

Perhaps pick him up and walk around your dark home, while gently jiggling him.

At this point he may stop crying, or he may continue crying. Continue walking around with him regardless of whether this actually soothes away his distress. Even if he continues to cry, there's at least an outside chance that the gentle jiggling is making him feel better. Or maybe it isn't. Or maybe it's at least helping *you* feel better, because now it seems like you're doing *something*. Anything.

(Have I mentioned you're exhausted?)

Fix #3: Try to soothe baby by nursing.

Try breastfeeding your baby again.

Go with one or two or all three of the above approaches.

You can cycle through all these potential fixes in the space of ten minutes or in the space of an hour. There's no need to pick one and stick with it. Go with one or two or all three as you see fit.

Again, just to be clear, at this point you're not trying to sleep-train your baby. He's too young to be left to cry until he falls back sleep.

And yet. There will be *some* crying involved.

This is where mothering is more art than science.

Your two- to six-week-old baby relies on you to have his needs met, but he also relies on you to give him a safe space for feeling and expressing a wide range of emotions. In the middle of the long, dark night, it's okay if your wee baby wails for two, five, or 20 minutes. It's okay to start allowing itty bitty increments of time to pass before momma swoops in to the rescue.

Responsive parenting doesn't mean that you're always jumping in to fix things. Sometimes, responsive parenting just involves *listening.* And right now, if you take a few minutes to listen, you'll hear that your baby is trying to tell you something along these lines: *We hang out as much as I want during the daytime. Why aren't we hanging out right now? Why the blazes do we have different rules for daytime and* *nighttime? This is outrageous! I think we'd all be better off if you just held me all night long. I *insist* on sleeping in your arms! I DEMAND to SPEAK with THE MANAGER!*

By allowing your baby to let you know that he's not really into separate sleep surfaces, you're honouring his right to communicate. You're honouring his developmental need to incrementally experience and deal with difficult feelings.

You're also honouring your own body's need for sleep by communicating the following back to your child: "Listen, Baby, if you wake up at night, of course I'll come and nurse you. But then I'm going to put you down. Because if I've already made the effort to nurse you to sleep, then I've done a good enough job. You can either take the sweet, soothing effect of my momma milk and fall asleep at my breast, or you can figure out how to fall asleep in the bassinet on your own after I've nursed you."

Consider it a battle of wills.[17] Who will win? Will baby end up sleeping in your bed or in your arms every night? Or will he be in the bassinet?

You decide, Momma.

All babies make it loudly, insistently known at some point in the first 40 days that they prefer to sleep in momma's arms—all night, every night. Whether or not you decide to adopt sleeping-in-arms at this point in the game will depend on your tolerance for nighttime crying.

This is where critics of anything that sounds *remotely* like a cry-it-out method usually act horrified, so let me be clear: Parents who allow for a little crying at night aren't cold or indifferent to their baby's needs; they're simply aware that a few, temporary nights of sniffles and snuffles at the newborn stage can prevent a lot more night-wakings (and concomitant tears) later on.

---

17   Do you find the notion of a nighttime "battle of wills" between a loving momma and her innocent little newborn a tad offensive? If so, no problem! It may be a sign that you're better off sharing a sleep surface. You do you.

Draw on your inner well of strength when your baby declares, "But I don't want to!"

If baby decides he doesn't like something—such as being put down in his bassinet at night, being placed in a baby carrier, hitching a ride in a car seat, or other routine aspects of baby life—you can acknowledge his feelings, but you don't necessarily have to change your plans. There's no need to give up on things you want baby to do just because he's stressed.

"Snowplow" and "helicopter" approaches to parenting took off with the generation who had their babies in the late 1990s, and they have remained popular in some parenting circles ever since. It started off innocently enough: Moms and dads were encouraged to always consider their children's feelings and to follow their child's lead. Baby, they were told, always knows best.

But both the snowplow approach (wherein parents plow all obstacles and causes of distress out of their baby's path) and the helicopter approach (wherein parents always hover nearby, ever vigilant, in case rescue is required) have arguably caused more problems for children than they've solved.

Clinicians, university administrators, and employers have all observed that higher numbers of people born since the 1990s have been reaching adulthood with relatively underdeveloped resilience, higher anxiety, and lower tolerance for stress, compared with previous generations. Levels of teen depression have risen, too. Psychiatrists caution that such things are never monocausal, but these worrying trends neatly line up with when snowplow and helicopter parenting approaches came on the scene.

Many aspects of responsive parenting are worth keeping, but the idea that parents should assume all responsibility for easing a child's distress needs to be unceremoniously retired. Empathy in our interactions with our children is essential, but consider this: it's also possible that you—*you* with your accumulated life wisdom and your higher functioning cerebral cortex—might be the one who knows best.[18]

If baby howls about something that has to happen (like being strapped into a car seat for a drive or getting less playtime with momma at night), keep at it. Be a good listener, sure, but stay strong and stand firm, Momma!

Tell your baby, "I'll be right back!"

There's something else I've been meaning to tell you: Your baby needs to occasionally spend time alone.

There's no need to *invent* reasons for leaving baby alone, but don't avoid opportunities to do so either. You are not obligated to be relentlessly present. If you need to step out of the room to shower or vacuum or return an email, put him in safe space,[19] and go.

Give him something interesting to look at (I mean an object, not Netflix) and let him amuse himself (or, as the case may be, let him be cranky by himself) for a moment without you hovering over him. You've got needs, too, and no one benefits if you completely ignore yours to attend to his.

When you leave your baby and head to another part of your home to work on mom stuff for a few minutes, don't forget to tell him where you're going and when you'll be back. Your baby won't yet understand what you're saying, of course, but this will set you up, right off the bat, with the good habit of sharing information with your child.

The risk of never, ever leaving your baby's side is that you increase the likelihood of acute separation anxiety. Some babies are biologically

---

18 I don't want to litter this book with too many sources—this isn't an academic treatise, after all—but I want to give a shout out to developmental psychologist Diana Baumrind's research on authoritative parenting, and to pediatrician and psychoanalyst D.W. Winnicott's notion of the "good-enough" parent. There's some good stuff there. Oldies but goldies, if you want to look them up.

19 Never leave baby unattended on an elevated surface such as a bouncy seat, table, high chair, chesterfield, or bed. If you step out of arm's reach, choose a safe location such as a crib, playpen, or blankie on the floor, away from pets.

more sensitive to separations, it's true, but parents can also create anxious babies fairly easily. Children who can't tolerate a moment apart from mom or dad can miss out on really wonderful experiences during their preschool years, like birthday parties and bouncy castles and swimming lessons!

The howling that can accompany drop-off attempts isn't easy on the child experiencing the distress, either. While every child experiences a certain amount of separation anxiety, acute versions of it are very uncomfortable for the child who is feeling upset.

You can reduce the risk of future intense separation anxiety by introducing itty-bitty alone times starting now. Learning how to be by himself in a safe environment for gradually increasing lengths of time is a skill that baby will strengthen with practice.

This is yet another aspect of motherhood where parenting is more of art than science. You want to create a warm bond with your baby. You want to establish a healthy level of attachment. But you also don't want to wait too long before beginning the very slow process of letting go.

Hold on, Momma, but not too tight.

Put the tiger in the tree.

Right around now, many babies get the "evening fussies."

Beginning at the age of two weeks, many babies begin to bob on and off the breast, appear unsettled, fuss, squirm, and—if you're really unlucky—wail uncontrollably for hours on end. To make things worse, the crying is often unsoothable. *Unsoothable* means mom and dad can't stop it, no matter what they do.

These, my friend, are the evening fussies.

And, get this: while the phenomenon *begins* around the age of two weeks, it then proceeds to get *worse* each night for about the next six to eight weeks. So keep in mind that, no matter how bad you had it today—tomorrow could be worse!

Fortunately, after peaking around the eight-week mark, the evening fussies tend to start decreasing in intensity. Between three and six months they usually dissipate altogether.

While the evening fussies are natural and expected, no one really knows why Mother Nature chose to punish bright-eyed, optimistic new parents with this confidence-wrecking racket.

Is colic caused by upset tummies? A temporary glitch in the development of the central nervous system? All manner of credentialed experts have been stymied in the quest for a definitive explanation.

I have my own (unqualified) theory why the evening/after-school/after-work fussies never really go away. I think it's because at about the 14-day mark babies become more conscious of the world around them and begin developing an internal monologue not unlike the one many of us have on our bus ride home at the end of the day. If your baby is screaming in the late afternoon and you're wondering what on earth is going on in his little head, I think it's something like this:

> I can't believe I said that to that other baby. Stupid. Stupid. Stupid… I hope that stranger in the supermarket didn't notice I smiled at him. I could've sworn he was my grandpa. How embarrassing! How come all of these old guys look alike?... I don't know if I'm ever going to figure out this whole talking thing. Just thinking about all those words—I'm going to hyperventilate… And am I the only one around here who hasn't figured out how to walk yet?

I solve my own evening fussies by reaching for a glass of red wine, but your baby has no outlet except raw rage.

The evening fussies usually take place near the end of the day.

For many babies, the evening fussies take place between about 6 and 9 pm, but there's a wide range of normal. At my workshops, I've heard of fussiness ramping up as early as noon and going strong as late as midnight. What kind of cockamamie definition of "evening" is that?!

No wonder some people find the baby stage *utterly* *intolerable*.

It may help you to know, however, that **noon to midnight** is generally the outside range of the evening-fussies period. **If you can't soothe away your baby's crying between midnight and noon**, it's probably a good idea to book a well-baby checkup with a medical professional, just to make sure that nothing else is going on.

> **Did you know?**
>
> Everyone notices the evening fussies, but not everyone notices that babies often exhibit the opposite behaviour in the morning. Between 6 and 9 am babies are most likely to either fall asleep or have quiet, alert time after breastfeeding.

Coping Strategies

If your baby has a case of the evening fussies, here are a dozen ideas to help you cope.

1: Recognize that this is normal baby behaviour.

Most babies have a regular evening fussy period, regardless of whether they're being raised by completely clueless parents or by the Mother of the Year. Some babies—some exceptional babies—will cry and cry and cry during the evening fussy period no matter what mom and dad try. If your baby is unsoothable in the late afternoons and/or evenings only, rest assured, it's not you—it's him!

Just knowing that this is expected and normal behaviour can often help parents power through this difficult time.

2: Try giving baby a soother.

Soothers aren't recommended during the first six weeks. That's because they work. Babies who use soothers sleep longer and nurse less, which interferes with establishing proper breastmilk supply in the first 40 days. And yet: if you have a baby with an aggravating case of the evening fussies, sometimes momma just needs a break. Using a soother might give you an hour or two of evening respite.

3: Try swaddling.

Again, sometimes a momma just needs a break from the crying.

4: Try a jiggling or rhythmic motion.

You know the drill.

5: Try the "tiger in a tree" hold.

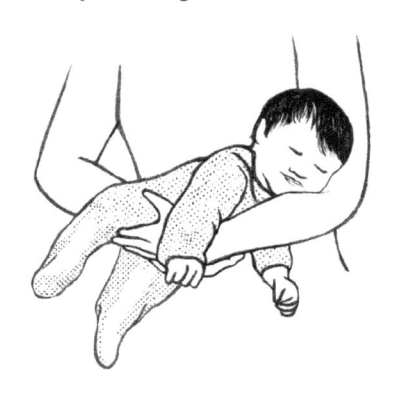

Rather than try to explain this hold with words, here's an illustration.[20]

There are a couple of key elements to mastering this hold.

First, part of the point is to put gentle pressure on baby's tummy. As long as your baby's neck is well supported, it's fine for baby to either face out (somewhat more upright) or to face down (like in the picture). And it's fine to either clasp both your arms together to support him or do this hold one-handed. Either way, just make sure there's a pressure point on your baby's tummy.

Secondly, there's a reason for holding him so that he lies on his left side as shown. People with upset tummies[21] tend to feel better if the opening from stomach to esophagus—which is toward our right side—faces up so that air has an easier time coming up and stomach contents are less likely to escape.

Still not working? Try a bit of gentle bouncing or dancing as you hold your tiger in his tree. Or walk around a bit—having something new to look at might distract your baby from the fussies.

With so much of infant care falling to momma, this is a great trick for dad to learn so he can pitch in. And then he can impress his friends and parents with his mad skills at soothing baby.

---

20   To find more visuals, google "magic baby hold" or "tiger in the tree hold."

21   Even if your baby's evening fussies aren't related to an upset tummy, the "tiger in the tree" hold will often still work.

6: Try breastfeeding again.

Many breastfed babies feed more often in the evening than in the morning. Experienced breastfeeding mothers know that the baby who was happily full for hours in the morning is often the same baby who wants to feed every hour, or half hour, or even continuously during the evening. This is normal feeding behaviour at this age and doesn't mean momma isn't making enough milk.

But if the bobbing-on-and-off thing is driving you nuts, don't be a martyr! Feel free to reach for a different tool in your toolbox.

7: Try close physical contact.

Put baby in a carrier and either walk around the house or outside. Better yet, if anyone has offered to help, get them to carry him around so you can get a break.

Sleep researcher Dr. James McKenna has come up with an interesting theory for why close physical contact might help. According to Dr. McKenna, up until the age of about one month, babies' breathing is involuntary and controlled by their brain stems, considered the brain's most primitive part. By the time they're seven months old, however, babies have typically mastered what Dr. McKenna calls "speech breathing," and are able to control the volume, tempo, and pitch of their cries.

Speech breathing is controlled by the brain's neocortex, which is responsible for executive functions, and comes so naturally that we never think about it: Human beings can talk without losing their breath. It's a fabulous bit of multitasking—to breathe and talk at the same time.

Dr. McKenna's theory is that the evening fussies might be a frustrating but harmless glitch in the development of speech breathing. Seen in this light, unstoppable crying is similar to an unshakable bout of hiccups.

Because speech breathing is a learned skill, acquired through hearing and feeling other people breathe, **Dr. McKenna posits that holding, carrying, and otherwise keeping young babies in close**

physical contact helps their neural networks develop more quickly and synchronously. So, although holding your baby close may not prevent or stop the inconsolable crying, it may at least reduce its severity and duration.

In other words, lots of holding and carrying could be the difference between the misery of mild fussing and the nerve-shattering shock of full-blown colic.

8: Try a brief sanity break.

Leave baby to cry someplace separate from you for a few minutes. You can put him down in a safe place, like his bassinet, and close the door and just walk away to take a bit of space for yourself.

Regroup.

Then go back.

9: Try acceptance.

Accept that baby will cry no matter what you try. I know your gut tells you that, if you're a good parent, merely holding your baby lovingly should be enough to stop crying.

But your gut is wrong.

The sweet, sweet embrace of your arms isn't enough.

Don't take your baby's sobbing personally. Even as he continues to cry, rest assured that he finds the physical contact with you reassuring.

10: There's no need for over-the-counter medications.

Over-the-counter medications are, generally speaking, ineffective marketing ploys designed to wrest money away from desperate parents.

11: Repeat to yourself, "There is nothing wrong with my breastmilk. There is nothing wrong with my breastmilk."

If you've got plenty of supply in the morning and your baby finds it delicious and filling, then it doesn't magically run out or go sour by the end of the day. Switching to formula or cutting your favourite foods out of your diet won't cure the fussies either. The intensity of your baby's cry is no more related to whether your baby is breast- or bottle-fed than it is to weather, political unrest, or crypto-currency fluctuations.

12: Mollycoddle with wild abandon.

If, mercifully, one of these suggestions works, you may get some well-meaning relative questioning your approach along the lines of: "It's nice that the breastfeeding/baby-carrier-wearing/tiger-in-the-tree-holding worked, but aren't you worried about mollycoddling? Isn't he going to manipulate you into constantly breastfeeding/baby-wearing/tiger-holding him from now until eternity and never move out of your house?"

Time for some reassurance. I can 100% guarantee that your baby will not be spoiled if you hold and nurse him often. In fact, studies have shown the opposite. The babies who are held a lot and responded to promptly are the babies who cry less. They cry less because they feel secure. A young child's need for his mother is very intense—as intense as his need for food. Filling that need will make your parenting job easier, not harder.

And, trust me, there's no way he'll want you to come anywhere near him by the time he's a tween anyway—especially not in public.

Oh, no, we've got to go through it!

While there are about a dozen different ways you can cope with the evening fussies, there's no definitive way to eliminate them entirely. As the characters say in Michael Rosen's bestselling children's book *We're Going on a Bear Hunt*, "We can't go over it, we can't go under it. Oh, no, we've got to go through it!"

The evening fussies are just one more thing that momma and daddy need to take in stride. They're part of the ups and downs of parenting. We've got to go through it.

CHAPTER 7:

Week 6 to Week 12

Introduce your baby to his public.

Congratulations—you've completed the babymoon phase!

In many cultures around the world, the babymoon phase ends around Day 40 (or, for babies born early, around five-and-a-half weeks after their original due date). After that, I'm pretty sure my peasant ancestors would go back to the fields to plant potatoes. But not you. You can go for a lunch date to show off your new baby to your old co-workers. You go, girl!

Starting at around one and a half months of age and for a few months after, babies are highly portable. This is a good time to make plans to see adult friends and do adult things with baby in tow.

It's also a great time to make new friends. Having a baby can expand your social networks. Take this opportunity to put yourself out there. Introduce yourself to a mom at your library's story time and ask her out to coffee. Strike up a conversation at the local park. Many of the parents you meet will never be more than passing acquaintances, but keep at it, and eventually you'll find your tribe.

Your *tribe*: Defined as the mommas who make you feel understood. The ones around whom you don't have to put on an act. The ones you can casually talk to about both your terrible and wonderful parenting experiences without feeling the need to insert caveats aimed at mollifying mothers who are better than you ("That's great that you read to your baby for a full half-hour *every day*") or appeasing mothers who are more clueless than you ("I'm sure your baby will turn out just *fine* without naps"). This fleeting phase of your life will be more interesting if you find some friends who really get you.

Meeting new people isn't just good for you—it's also great for your baby. Some days you'll feel like cocooning inside, which can be lovely. But your newborn is an instinctively social creature. If he doesn't get the occasional opportunity to experience chaos and noise, or to spend time around jumpy children and grumpy adults, he's at higher risk of being fearful of new people and experiences during his preschool years. It takes a village to raise a child.

So head out to the grocery store, invite moms for lattes—heck, invite moms for a pint, sign up for the community playgroup, check out story time at the library. The more you get out there, the more opportunities you'll create for different people to lean in, look your baby in the eye, and tell him how utterly adorable he is: "*Hey there, little fella, I like the cut of your jib!*"

Some of us grow up to be extroverts (those who get energized by being around other people), while some of us grow up to be introverts (those who refuel through quality alone time). Regardless of whether your baby ends up an introvert or an extrovert, he has a developmental need to figure out that his world is filled with men, women, children, pets, and wildlife of all temperaments, types, and sizes.

Pack in, pack out.

At this stage, most babies have six or more wet diapers each day, and some babies develop less frequent, but larger, bowel movements.

But where to toss that dirty diaper if baby *goes* when you're on the go?

Campgrounds and wilderness areas often have signs asking visitors to "pack in, pack out." Consider applying the same rule to your baby's stool. Your friends and family members will probably be too polite to say anything to you directly, but they *really* don't want your baby's poo-poo diaper fouling up their kitchen or bathroom waste receptacles. Strangers walking past public waste bins don't want to catch a whiff of that, either. So consider stocking your diaper kit with empty bags you can use to bring home your dirtiest diapers.

Figure out how to breastfeed in public.

Right about now most moms find that the challenges of the early weeks have worked themselves out and breastfeeding is a lot easier. If you're ready to take nursing to the next level, figuring out how to do it discreetly is a handy trick to learn at this stage.

One mom I met said she knew she'd nailed it the day she was at the car shop and a burly mechanic called her over to hand back her keys. She walked up to him, paid for the work, and asked a few questions about maintaining her vehicle. As he was about to take her out to the car, she said, "Just a minute, let me finish up."

"Finish up what?"

He hadn't realized that she'd been breastfeeding her baby throughout the entire interaction.

Breastfeeding is discreet when it's happening right next to you and you don't even notice.

Of course, learning to breastfeed discreetly is not a requirement. There are a couple of other ways to breastfeed in public, and if you prefer those, there's no harm, no foul. Again, you do you.

One non-discreet way to breastfeed in public is to just whip your shirt up or down and freely air your flesh. Sun's out, guns out.

The second non-discreet way to nurse is to use a nursing cover: a hot, giant, tent-like contraption that screams, "Hey, everyone!!! Look over here!!! Woman breastfeeding, with her boobies!!!"[22]

---

22 If you want a visual, there's a classic, 30-second Luvs diaper ad from 2013 that hilariously captures these first two approaches to public nursing: youtube.com/watch?v=B0oddLTdtD0. "She's already ordered." I love it!

Breastfeeding is the normal way to feed our babies, so to the mommas who breastfeed openly and without embarrassment: I salute you! But not every momma feels comfortable with overt public nursing. Fortunately, there's a third way to nurse in public, through discreet breastfeeding, or what some people call "the two-shirt method" or the "one-up-one-down method." Let me tell you how it's done.

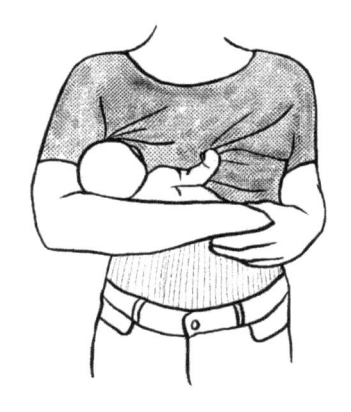

To start, you'll want to wear a **double-layered** outfit. The **inside** layer (the underneath layer) should be low-cut enough that you can pull it under your breast when you're ready to nurse. The **top** layer can be whatever you want to wear.

You can buy purpose-made clothes with nursing slits, but these garments often create a larger opening than you need, and set you up for the risk of unwanted exposure. The easiest—and cheapest—route is to simply dig through the slaying wardrobe you already own and find two layers.

It's easier to be discreet if the inner layer is the same colour as the outer layer, but this isn't necessary.

When you're ready to nurse, silently unsnap your nursing bra.

CLICK!

(*Ok, maybe that wasn't so subtle.*)

If you use breast pads,[23] find an out-of-sight spot to put them—don't just flop them down on the table for everyone to ogle.

Next, bring your baby's face in, level with your breast. This is the opposite of what you would do in private. In private you probably bring in baby's face as the last step, but in public you'll want to bring

---

23 Nursing pads are handy for moms who make so much milk that they leak. Consider acquiring a pair of woolen pads. They don't get damp like cotton, and they don't feel as menstrual-pad-on-my-breast-sweaty as the disposable ones. Best of all, you only need to wash them about once per month. Seriously. Once per month. Wool is pretty amazing.

baby in earlier, before the opening is ready. His head will block the last bit of the operation from public view.

Next, stick your hand under just your **outer** shirt and—now that you're in there—subtly manoeuvre your **inner** layer down and out of the way, so there's a clear path to your breast. No one can see you doing this because your hand is covered by your outer shirt. Now the only thing between your baby and your breast is your outer clothing layer.

Next is the tricky part—the part you'll want to practise in front of a mirror. One of your hands is holding baby in position. This leaves your remaining hand to complete the process. In a quick, slick, single-handed move—with your baby facing your breast and blocking the view—lift up your outer layer with your thumb, hold down the inner layer with a couple of other fingers, and latch your baby.

This last step—the part where you latch your baby—can be challenging if you feel you don't have enough privacy, because there may be a split second where some flesh is exposed. If you find yourself in a situation where all eyes

> **Did you know?**
>
> One of the predictors of whether a mother will breastfeed for at least six months is how comfortable she is breastfeeding with family and friends around.

seem to be upon you, one option is to wait for a natural opportunity, like when your mates are distracted (perhaps by the arrival of another guest or by a riveting story being told at the other end of the table). Another option is to create a temporary barrier. Turn away, latch, and then turn back to the conversation. Or flip a flowy scarf over baby for just the second or two it takes to get him going.

Once your baby is latched, no one will see any unexpected parts of your body.

No one will see the top of your breast—which is still covered by your outer shirt. No one will see your ribs, side, or flabby post-baby belly[24]—those are still covered by your inner shirt. No one will see your breast or nipple—which is covered by baby himself. And here's the best part: If your baby unexpectedly whips his head away, your outer layer will immediately drop and cascade over your breast.

The vast majority of people walking by will simply assume that you're holding your baby—and that he's sleeping with his face buried against you. The only ones who'll realize you're breastfeeding are other mommas who've figured out how to nurse discreetly too.

Once you've figure out how to comfortably nurse in public, the world's your oyster. You can now nurse your darling anywhere, anytime. How liberating![25]

Another tip to make public breastfeeding easier: Nurse before you go out.

Offer to fill up your baby's tank before leaving home. This buys you time to get settled wherever you're going before you have to nurse again.

Once you arrive at your destination, nurse at the first sign of hunger. If you wait, hoping he'll change his mind, he may grow increasingly upset. Soon all eyes will be on the screaming baby. You're going to feel hot and flustered and it'll be much harder to latch inconspicuously.

Moms who are out and about sometimes end up nursing their baby more frequently than they would at home, just to keep baby content and quiet.

---

[24] If you're a celebrity, you may be unfamiliar with "flabby post-baby belly." It's what the rest of us look like around the midriff for roughly the two decades it takes our bodies to recover from having a baby.

[25] If you're willing to look past the 1977 low-definition picture quality, a vintage Sesame Street clip shows singer-songwriter Buffy Sainte-Marie discreetly breastfeeding her son Dakota "Cody" Starblanket Wolfchild on network television: youtube.com/watch?v=l2RwZW2j3-U. It's sweet, simple, and just under a minute long.

Alternatively, if you're looking for more of a "how to," you can find YouTube tutorials by googling "two-shirt nursing" or "one-up-one-down breastfeeding."

Always ask for permission before feeding your baby in public.

Ha, I'm just messing with you.

Obviously, there's no need to announce that you're about to breastfeed. If you bring attention to what you're about to do, it'll be much harder to be inconspicuous. Simply proceed to feed your child at your breast as if it were the most normal thing in the world, which, of course, it is. Your matter-of-fact attitude in this situation will put others at ease.

People eat. (And usually not in bathrooms.) It's no big deal.

Do let your baby use you like a soother.

Many babies develop a somewhat predictable nursing pattern at this age, but don't just go by the clock. Nurse whenever your baby is unsettled, even if you just nursed him 10 minutes ago, because babies have a biological need to be nursed on demand during their waking hours until around the one-year mark.

Breastfeeding on demand throughout baby's first year isn't just something you do to provide him with food. Your baby breastfeeds for many reasons other than hunger.

He breastfeeds because he likes the feeling of security it gives him; the feeling that there are people he can trust to keep him comfortable and safe. He does it because he finds the sound of your heartbeat soothing. He does it because he needs to satisfy his sucking instincts. Breastfeeding is how he first communicates with you, and you with him.

Right around now a well-meaning friend might advise you to unlatch your baby because "he's just using you as a soother." The proper response to this is: "I know, Felicia! Isn't that awesome? It's like I have a new superpower!"

Using mom as a pacifier is exactly how breastfeeding is meant to work. Nursing pacifies your baby, comforts him, reassures him, relaxes him, and puts him to sleep. As a mother, it gives you self-confidence when you know what to do to keep your baby content. If you offer your breast only as food and never as a pacifier, you'll miss out on one of the best tools you have for making this whole parenting thing as easy as possible. Nursing keeps your baby well fed *and* happy. There's no reason to hold back.

Expect your breasts to feel a lot less full.

Now that milk production is established and the hormones of childbirth have decreased, most moms find their breasts begin to feel softer. If your breasts suddenly begin to feel "empty," it's not because you've run out of milk—it's because your body has finally figured out what it's doing.

Clever body![26]

Along with the softer breasts, many moms find that breastfeeding becomes less time-consuming and intense around the six-week mark. It's not unusual for a baby of this age to feed for just two to ten minutes at each nursing. But reduced time at the breast doesn't mean he's getting less milk—your body is now producing 500 to 700 calories of milk a day—it just means that your clever little baboo has figured out how to guzzle down those calories quickly. As long as your baby continues to gain weight at the normal rate, less time at the breast is just fine.

Many babies also begin spacing their feedings further apart at this stage, and some even begin developing a somewhat more predictable nursing pattern. In other words, some moms will notice that their two-month-old tends to breastfeed at certain times of day.

Just to be clear, both of these (the shorter feedings and the emerging feeding schedule) are baby-led developments. Your baby is 100% in charge of making breastfeeding more efficient, just as he's 100% in charge of becoming more efficient with his bowel movements (you may notice that you're finally cutting back on the ten-diaper-a-day

---

[26] Not really. If our bodies were truly clever, our post-baby bellies would shrink first, and the fuller breasts would last for at least one swimsuit season.

habit you had during the newborn stage). Your baby reaches these milestones at his own pace, and there's no rush to get there.

Give your baby tummy time.

Now that your babymoon is over, remember to give your baby some daily, supervised tummy time on a blanket when he's awake. Tummy time on a blanket helps your growing baby to:

- ✓ Strengthen the muscles in his neck, shoulders, and back
- ✓ Develop head control
- ✓ Develop arm reach
- ✓ Learn to roll over, and
- ✓ Learn to crawl.

At first, your baby will fuss because he won't have the muscle strength to be comfortable in this position. You can follow his lead and keep the first few blanket adventures quite short. But day by day he'll grow stronger and enjoy his tummy playtime more and more.

You can put some fun items on the blanket—they don't have to be toys; they just have to be safe for baby to put in his mouth.

Many moms also put at least one interesting object just out of reach, because babies (like all people) like having something to strive for.

Keep putting baby down for daytime naps.

Throughout their first three or four months, babies can sleep anywhere, any time during the day. There is no predictability to their sleep.

What you'll find between Week 6 and Week 12, though, is that the daytime naps generally start getting shorter and more spread out. Babies also start experiencing longer periods of wakefulness. The longest stretch of wakefulness happens at the end of the day and can last as long three hours, thanks to baby's developing circadian rhythm.

These developments are baby-led, which means that there is nothing mom and dad need to do to increase baby's daytime wakefulness.

While naps naturally tend to get more spread out at this age, many moms find that baby is less prone to fussing if they embark on a soothing-to-sleep routine after one to two hours of wakefulness throughout the day—starting from when baby is up for the day to sometime in the late afternoon.

If baby doesn't fall asleep, that's fine. It's giving him the *opportunity* for a nap that counts. At this age, babies still find it hard to be awake for much more than two hours at a time before about 4 or 5 pm, and as mom and baby get busier during the day it can get harder to notice sleepy signs. You can hedge your bets by *offering* to soothe your baby to sleep after about one to two hours of wakefulness throughout the day.

Watch for baby to make night bedtime earlier.

If your newborn was falling asleep for the night between 9 pm and midnight, sometime around two months old he'll naturally begin to adopt an earlier bedtime, likely between about **8 and 11 pm**. Follow your baby's lead and watch for his signs of drowsiness to start coming earlier. If you miss his glazed-over eyes, turning head, slowed movements, and yawning, then your baby could become overtired, then wired, and then stay up waaaay past when you were planning to hit the hay.

You can try partial night-weaning now, if you like.

Nursing on demand remains important during the daytime.

Nursing on demand is still very important during the *daytime* at this age. After 4 am, there's no point in making baby wait even a minute for a feeding.

That's right: 4 am. Daytime begins around 4 or 5 am, according to young babies, even if parents find this definition of "daytime" inhumane. The majority of babies are biologically wired at this age to need food around this time. So, starting about 4 am, and for all the daytime hours until he turns in for the night (at a bedtime of his own choosing), everything will go a lot smoother if you simply nurse him, pronto, as soon as he wants to.

In fact, you *want* baby to wake up by about 5 am, because at that early hour there's a decent chance you can nurse him *back* to sleep and then return to bed for a nice sleep-in yourself. If you're lucky and do manage to nurse him back to sleep, the two of you might not get up again until 8:30 or 9 am, which will make you feel like a new woman.

If he waits until shortly after 6 am to wake up, it'll be much harder to nurse him back to sleep, and the two of you may be up for the day. At 6 am. *Ugh*.

Nursing on demand remains important during the day, but it no longer needs to be "on demand" throughout the entire night.

Your baby may now be ready for a momentous milestone: Lengthening his nighttime sleep.

"Ready" is a tricky concept. Let's be honest—he may be physically ready, but he's probably not keen. He'd probably *prefer* for you to continue to nurse him on demand throughout the night. But chances are that *you*, Momma, would prefer to get a little more restorative sleep each night. If that's the case, all you need to get baby on board is a little night-weaning.

A little night-weaning is all it takes and then—easy-peasy-lemon-squeezy—your baby will be sleeping through the night in no time!

Well, okay, maybe not quite "through" the night.

At this age we're talking about *partial* night-weaning, because you only have about a **four- to six-hour** window to work with. On top of that, your baby might be going to bed as late as midnight (which is way past when you were planning to turn in) and getting up as early as 4 am (which is well before you were planning to be up); so, let's just drop this whole charade of sleeping "through" the night right now. What we're really talking about between Week 6 and Week 12 is *lengthening* his longest stretch of nighttime sleep.

So, uh, what does "lengthening" night sleep mean, exactly?

If you haven't done any partial night-weaning yet, your baby likely falls asleep for the night between 9 and 11 pm (or as late as midnight), and then gets up to nurse *several* times throughout the night—sometimes waking as often as every couple of hours. Some babies are then up for the day starting at around 4 or 5 am, while others can keep nursing back to sleep until 8 or 9 am.

Once you've *completed* the partial night-weaning, your baby will be able to sleep for *at least* a four- to six-hour stretch at night. Some babies will sleep for even longer stretches after partial weaning. It depends on the individual baby. Some have a physiological need to eat every four to six hours at this age. Others don't. And since there's no external test that can tell you which category your baby falls into, **the ultimate result of your partial night-weaning** will be a *surprise*. (*Don't you love surprises!?*)

It will, however, be one of the following **five** sleep-length patterns:

- ✓ **One nursing before 4 am, and then up and at 'em.** If you have a baby who can't go longer than four to six hours without nursing at night and who has trouble falling back asleep during the early-morning nursing, the end result of partial weaning will be that baby falls asleep at **his self-selected bedtime**, then wakes up once between 9 pm and 4 am to nurse back to sleep, then wakes up again to nurse around 4 or 5 am, and then *stays up* at that early morning hour. In other words, your baby will have just one night nursing after you complete the partial night-weaning, but over the course of a night that ends quite early.

- ✓ **One nursing before 4 am, and then one last chunk of night-sleep after the early morning nursing.** In this scenario, the end result of partial night-weaning will be that baby wakes up once between 9 pm and 4 am to nurse back to sleep, and then wakes up again around 4 or 5 am to nurse back down for a little more night sleep. In other words, your baby will have two "night" nursings, but over the course of a *longer* night.

- ✓ **Zero nursing before 4 am, but then up and at 'em.** If you have a baby who can go 7–9 hours without nursing at night but who has trouble falling back asleep during the early morning nursing, the result of your efforts will be that baby sleeps through until around 4 or 5 am, then wakes up to nurse at that hour and stays up to seize the day. *Carpe diem* indeed.

- ✓ **Zero nursing before 4 am, and then one last chunk of night-sleep after the early-morning nursing.** In this scenario, baby sleeps through until around 4 or 5 am, then wakes up to nurse at that hour, and then falls back asleep for a little more night sleep.

- ✓ **The full-meal deal.** *Ooooh. Yeaaaah.* Baby not only has no physiological need for a middle-of-the-night feeding—he also eliminates the 4 or 5 am nursing on his own. Result for momma: seven to eight hours of uninterrupted sleep!

Just to reiterate: **Momma** decides whether or not to do partial night-weaning to lengthen baby's night sleep, but **Baby** gets to decide which of the five sleep-length scenarios the family ends up with after partial night-weaning.

Sleeping through the night is a brain milestone—not a feeding milestone.

Human beings of all ages experience sleep-wake rhythms every night. Even you!

The difference between an adult (at least one who doesn't suffer from insomnia[27]) and a baby is that the adult's brain long ago figured

---

[27] Insomnia means taking more than 30 minutes to fall asleep, waking up during the night for more than 30 minutes, or waking up 30 minutes earlier than you intended to.

out how to ride the sleep wave back into slumber—often without fully awakening. A *newborn* baby's brain, however, mostly relies on the soothing effects of nursing and suckling to catch that sleep wave.

Partial night-weaning is just a momma's way of stepping out of the way and allowing the brain of her no-longer-newborn baby to learn new ways of riding the sleep wave back into slumber.

Some would-be sages may suggest topping up a baby's tank before bedtime with some rice cereal or a bottle of formula, but this advice is misguided. The formula or cereal will just cut down on the amount of breastmilk baby takes in, and do nothing for baby's sleep.

If we could eat our way into 11 hours of uninterrupted sleep, then you'd never hear of a mom with a baby older than six months complain about night-waking. After all, kids over six months old are eating solids. But if a child hasn't been night-weaned, he'll continue waking up throughout the night for his milkie, even if he had a steak dinner right before bed.

In other words, being a good sleeper is primarily a brain thing, and not a belly thing.

Partial night-weaning is all about your sleep intake, Momma.

Some parents assume, incorrectly, that the purpose of night-weaning is to reduce baby's nighttime breastmilk intake. But no.

The only reason to night-wean is this:

> Momma.
>
> Needs.
>
> More.
>
> Sleep.

That's it. That's the bottom line.

So if you end up decreasing baby's nighttime breastfeeding without increasing *your* nighttime sleeping, then you still haven't solved the problem.

It's natural for parents to gravitate towards gentle, no-cry methods of easing their babies away from nighttime milkie. Too often, however, parents who try no-cry approaches end up stuck in a rut of constantly soothing their babies back to sleep. If you're holding your baby for hours in the middle of the night or repeatedly popping the soother back into his mouth to get him to settle, then he's been night-weaned off breastmilk, sure, but he hasn't been night-weaned off momma.

If you replace the nighttime breastfeeding with other parent-led soothing methods, then you haven't actually night-weaned.

Wait, did you just say "crying"? Nuh, uh. Not gonna happen. I'm not that kind of momma.

Night-weaning isn't for everyone, and that's okay.

If you want to avoid night-weaning while maximizing nighttime sleep, then bed-sharing may be the best approach for your family. When baby shares a bed with momma, it's easy to nurse while he and mom are both in a light-sleep state, which means less sleep fragmentation for everybody.

But if momma is ready for a little more nighttime shut-eye and she's *not* co-sleeping with her baby, then there's only one way to get there: night-weaning. And if you are night-weaning, then I need to level with you, my friend: there *will* be crying.

But there's a book out there called the *No Cry Sleep Solution*! I'm going to run out and buy it.

Catchy title, for sure. But this book is actually about how to do lots and lots of soothing while baby is night-weaning. Why lots of soothing? Because baby is crying. There is still crying involved.

Well, I just googled "sleep," "baby," and the name of my city, and I found about a dozen accredited sleep consultants who offer gentle, no-cry sleep coaching.

There are all sorts of variations on night-weaning out there: no-cry, gentle-cry, spaced-cry, graduated-cry, check-and-console, and extinction (aka, the oft-maligned "cry-it-out" approach). No matter what it's called, there is always crying involved. It's the soothing that differentiates the various approaches—lots of soothing, some soothing, no soothing—not the crying.

There's nothing intrinsically better or worse *for baby* in each approach—they're just different. And the differences include these two variables: efficacy and degree of difficulty. The more soothing is involved, the more nights of crying you have to endure. And the more nights of crying you have to endure, the more likely you are to throw in the towel and give up.

Whether they're charging $100 for a short consult or $1,000 for a full package, the sleep consultants accredited by Genuine Accredited Sleep Institutes™ earn their keep by coaching parents and doing lots of handholding through the difficult process of crying and soothing. If a $1,000 accredited sleep coach is what you need to get through the sleep-training night, then go for it.[28]

Just be aware that there will still be crying involved in the process.

Signs of readiness in momma

Once baby is old enough for partial night-weaning (so: right about now), the decision about when to start depends almost entirely on whether momma (rather than baby) is showing signs of readiness.

You've been running on half a tank of gas since baby was born—and probably more or less handling the shocking loss of restorative sleep—but rumour has it that most moms experience peak exhaustion sometime between 40 days and three months postpartum. So if you feel like you haven't done a good job handling the fractured sleep so far, then consider this: you're about to feel a lot worse. It's as if that post-birth adrenaline has finally worn off, and now your body and mind are fading fast. Every fibre of your being begs for mercy. *Enough already.*

---

[28] I'm serious. If a sleep coach or consultant helps you through this difficult period, then hire one. If you're not getting the support you need from family or friends, then you need to find another buddy to talk to. A paid sleep consultant can be that buddy. Having someone who can help you find answers to your questions will give you the confidence you need to move toward your dream of more sleep for the whole family.

Signs that you're ready for partial night-weaning:

✓ Weepiness.

✓ Irritability.

✓ Escalating impatience for the demands of your older children.

✓ Complete intolerance for the shortcomings of your spouse.

✓ Fogginess.

✓ Grogginess.

✓ Utter exhaustion.

But you may be thinking: Isn't it selfish for a mother to put her need for sleep ahead of her helpless baby's cries?

Of course not! There's nothing selfish about getting the sleep you need to function as the kind of parent you always wanted to be: patient, kind, and with a zest for fun. The whole family will benefit from a momma who's physically and emotionally healthy. Has anyone ever told you, "You know, you really should aim to get *less* sleep"?

I didn't think so.

Also, keep in mind that better nighttime sleep isn't just for *your* benefit. It's for baby's benefit, too. Babies are also less testy and weepy in the day if they've had a good rest at night.

That being said, if you *aren't* ready to night-wean, then there's no need to do it at this stage.

Now is when nature presents you with the earliest and simplest opportunity for lengthening your baby's night sleep, but you can wait as long as you want to night-wean, because this is your family and you know how much sleep you need. Don't let other people's expectations push you into it if you're not ready.

Why baby may be ready to start night-weaning now

Since *newborns* need to be nursed on demand 24/7, you may be wondering what changes have occurred to make partial night-weaning an option for your growing baby now. Here are some milestones that occur at this stage:

- ✓ **Mom reaches peak milk production**, which means that nursing throughout the *entire* night is no longer essential to establishing or maintaining an adequate milk supply.

- ✓ **Baby becomes more efficient at breastfeeding**, which means he's got the skills to meet all of his nutritional needs in, say, an 18-hour rather than a 24-hour window.

- ✓ **Baby stops pooping at night**, his first milestone on the way to being fully toilet-trained one day! He's no longer experiencing the rousing effects of having a full-blown bowel movement in the middle of the night.

- ✓ **The evening fussies reach their peak.** Starting between six and eight weeks of age, the evening fussies begin decreasing in intensity every night. You've finally turned the corner: no matter how bad you had it this evening, tomorrow should be *better!*

- ✓ **Your baby's body temperature begins to take a bigger dip at night**, which sets the stage for longer sleep periods.

- ✓ **Day/night confusion is ending.** This is the age at which your baby starts figuring out that there's a daytime and a nighttime, and that more of the sleep stuff happens at night. As a result, the longest single sleep period begins to predictably occur in the evening hours.

- ✓ **Your baby's developing brain is making more neural connections**, and becomes capable of figuring out new ways of riding the normal sleep-wake cycles back into slumber.

All that being said, though, there's no single, universally accepted method for determining *when* a baby is physically and developmentally ready for partial night-weaning.

For obvious ethical and legal reasons, it's impossible to do human research at a population level in a lab where all complicating factors are controlled. So there's no legal, ethical way to *scientifically* prove when a baby is ready for night weaning or sleep training. There's also no legal, ethical way to scientifically prove how much crying is too much crying.

What we do know is this: Public health researchers are focused on risk-reduction and the interpretation of biological processes. Their job is to look for harm in the name of health. Through this lens, the social and cultural environment in which a baby is raised doesn't track. Public health researchers aren't asking how your healthy great-grandmother got her healthy babies to sleep through the night; public health researchers ask whether a baby's stress hormones are elevated when he cries (yes, yes they are, in that all humans of all ages experience elevated stress hormones when we cry) and they ask whether there is an association between negligent parenting and crying (yes, yes there is, in that negligent parenting is defined by a long-term, chronic failure to respond to a baby's needs in a loving and appropriate way). Public health researchers take these two known factors—elevated stress hormones and narrowly selected evidence from a cohort representing one extreme sub-set of the parenting population—and have used these as a basis for generalized recommendations that, since the 1990s, have been depriving generations of mommas of the sleep we need.

To clarify: I am not an anti-public health zealot. I love public health recommendations! I try to drink less, walk more and keep my hands away from my T-zone, all thanks to the good advice imparted by public-health researchers. I'm just wary when extremely limited data is used as the basis for excessive and patronizing recommendations that take common sense out of raising a baby. And this despite the robust research around how a good night's sleep can contribute to good health and longevity!

The current stigma around sleep training is based on a dismally narrow understanding of how night weaning and sleep training actually work in real life with real individuals. Sorry, science: Not good enough. I'm going to go with the collective wisdom of mommas on this one.

So, what do mommas using momma ways of knowing (not scientists using reductionist ways of knowing) have to say about *when* a baby is physically and developmentally ready for partial night-weaning?

Generally, most moms agree it's easier if you wait until the *peak* of the evening fussies has passed before embarking on any night-weaning efforts. But if your baby never really experienced the evening fussies, or if he seems to be on a downward trajectory from the peak of inconsolable fussing and crying…Well, it's not science, right? So the jury's out on the best time to start.

Some moms say you can get a healthy baby to sleep through a four- to six-hour stretch at night starting when he's five to six weeks old (or five to six weeks after the original due date for babies born early). This is generally around the 40-day mark. Other moms say night-weaning at two months or nine weeks is the ticket. Other moms say to wait until baby weighs at least 11 or 12 pounds.

Other mommas believe only a sociopath would force an itty-bitty baby to do any amount of forced night-weaning at any age.

Use ***your own*** judgment.

If health professionals are satisfied with your baby's weight gain and growth, and if you feel breastfeeding is going well, then at some point between the ages of 40 days and three months you can choose to join the many mommas who decide to lengthen their baby's night sleep.

I've seen the night light! Sign me up. It's go time!

Okay, let's ease into night-weaning by breaking it up into three chunks.

Phase 1: Night-wean for a three-hour period, during the first half of the night.

When your baby falls asleep for the night, note the time and then add three hours. For example, if your baby falls asleep at 10 pm, then write down 10 pm to 1 am on a sheet of paper. This will be your three-hour window for tonight.

During these three hours, regardless of whether your baby is sleeping soundly or awake and crying, you won't go in to nurse him. If he wakes up at 12:05 am, you won't nurse him until 1 am. If he wakes up at 12:45 am, you won't nurse him until 1 am.

Outside of those hours, however, you continue your normal practice of nursing on demand. In other words, if your baby is sleeping at 1 am (because he slept straight through from 10 pm to 1 am, or because he woke up, cried, and fell back asleep), you'll let him continue sleeping. But as soon as he wakes up after this arbitrary 1 am mark, you'll nurse him.

Truly, it is not unreasonable for a healthy baby more than 40 days old to give momma a rest for a three-hour period.

Try night-weaning for a three-hour period, **starting the clock at baby's slightly different, *baby-selected* bedtime each night**, and see how it works out. In the majority of cases, the length and intensity of baby's crying **will begin diminishing after a few days, and will decrease significantly after about five nights**. If this isn't how it plays out at your house, then use your judgment to decide whether to abandon night-weaning for now. Maybe you need to wait a few more weeks before tackling it again.

But if all goes well, you can try lengthening your sleep period by moving on to Phase 2.

Phase 2: Lengthen night-weaning to a four-hour period, still during the first half of the night.

If everything is going well after you night-weaned for a three-hour period during the first half of the night, then once you're ready—perhaps in a day, perhaps in a week—try night-weaning for a four-hour period.

Again, use **baby's self-selected** bedtime to time each night's sleep-training period. Depending on when your baby decides to fall asleep for the night, the sleep-training period could end up being 8 pm to midnight, 9 pm to 1 am, 10 pm to 2 am, 11 pm to 3 am, or any range in-between. Make sure to always write down the end time, because in the middle of the night—with a baby crying—parents tend to second-guess the plan if it's not on paper.

Phase 3: Night-wean baby to 4 or 5 am during the second half of the night.

For babies between the ages of 40 days and four months, four hours seems to be the outer limit for parent-led night-weaning, but there's more than one four-hour chunk of time in a typical night.

After your baby has mastered sleeping a minimum of four hours straight during the *first* half of the night, you can tackle the *second* half of the night.

What you do is this: When your baby awakens <u>after a minimum of four hours of sleep during the first half of the night</u>, get him back to sleep with a nice, long, languorous middle-of-the-night breastfeeding session. Once he's asleep, put him down in his bassinet or crib, and <u>then wait until at least **4 am**</u> before nursing him again.

That's it. Your part is done!

Now you can sit back and see which of the five sleep-length scenarios (the ones described a few pages back) you end up with.

This is the part where *baby-led* night-weaning takes over.

As mentioned, two four-hour chunks from baby's self-selected bedtime to about 4 or 5 am constitute the outer limit for **parent-led** partial night-weaning, but there's also such a thing as **baby-led** night-weaning.

Many moms find that if they start with partial night-weaning during the first half of the night, their baby ends up lengthening the rest of his night sleep on his own.

This is amazing, but true.

You're not the only fan of uninterrupted sleep—your baby might like it, too, once he tries it! Once you help your baby acquire this new superpower—of riding the wave back to sleep without milkie—there's a decent chance he'll figure out on his own how to lengthen the rest of his night sleep, from three hours to five hours, seven hours, or more.

And if your baby doesn't decide on his own to lengthen the rest of his night sleep past two four-hour chunks, then try to be grateful that you're getting a little bit more uninterrupted sleep than in the newborn stage. Some babies have a physiological need to nurse once between bedtime and 4 am, while others don't. Both behaviours are within the range of normal.

If you have one of those babies who can't sleep more than four to six hours at a stretch at this age, you can take heart in the knowledge that **at nine months** you'll have another opportunity to encourage your baby to lengthen his night sleep.

Night-weaning is *not* easy.

Night-weaning involves crying, often for hours, and no mother likes to hear her baby cry. Listening to a baby cry without going to him goes against your instincts and takes tremendous fortitude. It's especially hard when you know you have a sure-fire way to end your baby's distress. You could just go in and nurse him and the crying would be over in less than a minute.

> "Today Anthony turned seven weeks old and he's now falling asleep every night between about 10 pm and midnight, and sleeping through the night until between about 5 am and 7 am. And this without any night-weaning at all! Avery and Ben never did that. We had to go through hours of crying with them, and it was painful. I'd always thought moms who said stuff like this were exaggerating, but he really has done this. He started sleeping through the night with no crying or night-weaning. Is it because he is a different baby? Or is it because there is something different about our parenting? I guess I'll never know!"
>
> —Mom of three

This is why there's no point in letting your baby tackle this developmental milestone unless you're truly ready. Partial night-weaning is hard enough already. It's essentially impossible if Mom's heart isn't in it.

Night-weaning is incredibly simple.

Night-weaning is incredibly hard, but at the same time incredibly simple. If you don't want to nurse your baby at night, then don't nurse your baby at night.

That's worth saying twice, because it's so simple, yet it eludes so many: If you do not want to nurse your baby at night then what you need to do is not nurse your baby at night. That's it. That's really all there is to it.

This is what the sleep coaches are paid to tell you.

The challenge, of course, is that if you don't nurse baby at night, he is going to cry. And cry. And cry some more. So, what do you do when baby wakes up to nurse?

You have two options.

One option is to just leave baby to cry until he drifts off to sleep. This can take hours. Each night. For four or five nights.

Another option is to try to soothe baby while he cries himself to sleep. In other words, lots of rocking and walking and belly rubbing. This can take even more hours. Over even more nights. Over several weeks, even.

Both options involve tears, both yours and your baby's.

But in the end you'll achieve the holy grail of a good night's rest, for everybody.

Just imagine how much you could get done in your day if you started to get enough sleep again![29]

A few more notes on partial night-weaning….

---

29 Answer: Preside over the affairs of an entire nation? Jacinda Ardern was prime minister of New Zealand from October 2017 to January 2023 and gave birth to a baby girl while in office. That means she was doing everything you're doing *while also running the whole damn country.* I don't know how she organized her nighttime parenting back in the baby stage (none of my business), but presumably sleep would help with both parenting and governing a nation.

What's normal for crying? How do I know when to intervene?

There aren't any rules here, so you'll have to listen to your mom gut. The best information I can pass on (from other moms who've been there before you) is:

- If your baby carries on crying really intensely or powerfully for 15 or 20 minutes without stopping and then settles, that's fine.

- If the cry is lower pitched than a panicked or pained crying, then you don't need to worry.

- If the tone says he's mad or sad, let him process those strong feelings. They're *his* feelings, and he has a right to feel them. If you hear a cry that says, "I'm absolutely terrified," though, you'll want to step in and save him.

- If the crying is really intense for five or ten minutes, then there's a lull, then baby gets worked up again, then stops again—in other words, if the crying comes in little peaks—and your baby does it for an hour or two, the moms who've been there before say: don't worry about it.

Parent-led night-weaning can't go much past 4 am.

Babies can't cry themselves back to nighttime sleep after about 4 or 5 am. After 4 am you can *try* to nurse baby back to sleep, but if he doesn't doze off then you'll probably have to get up for the day with him. Baby gets to make the call after 4 am.

No harm done.

Contrary to the fear-mongering of some soi-disant experts, you will not traumatize your baby by leaving him to cry until he drifts off to sleep. Your baby will greet you with his usual cheery smile the morning after a night-weaning session.

In his classic book *Healthy Sleep Habits, Happy Child*, pediatric sleep expert Dr. Marc Weissbluth theorizes that the reason babies seem unperturbed by night-weaning or sleep-training is because the crying is taking place during a biological sleep mode. Your baby is already in the foggy groggy zone.

If you were to leave your baby crying during his biological awake time (which you wouldn't, because you're a good momma), on the other hand, it would be quite distressing for him. Plus, your baby wouldn't fall asleep if you left him to cry during a biological awake time because, as Dr. Weissbluth points out, while you can force a person awake, you can't force a person asleep.

But when your baby is in a semi-alert sleepy mode, it's entirely possible that his brain processes a crying episode in a different manner.

A baby who can count on his parents' loving attention during wakeful periods can handle a few exceptional nights of sleep-time crying. The crying is tougher on parents than it is on the child.

Honestly, I can't emphasize this enough—no harm done.

One popular argument against sleep-training goes along the following lines: It would be distressing for an adult to cry themselves to sleep each night, and the same is true for a wee baby calling out for his parents in the only way he can. Really pulls on the old heartstrings! And it truly would be horrifying if someone had to cry themselves to sleep *every* night.

The missing piece here is that babies who are night-weaned do *not* cry themselves to sleep **every** night.

Babies who are night-weaned typically experience **four to five nights** of crying before they drift off to sleep, and after that they naturally, biologically, organically figure out how to ride the sleep wave—without the whole crying bit.

To soothe or not to soothe? Either way there will be crying.

Mom and dad get to choose whether they prefer to night-wean with no soothing or lots of soothing. Some parents want to feel like they're doing something, anything, during this difficult process, so they choose to do lots of soothing, while other parents want to get the whole business over with as soon as possible, so they choose no soothing. It's an individual choice.

Just one small consideration—when parents approach night-weaning with lots of soothing, it tends to prolong the process. In other words, you'll be working on sleep-training for more hours over more nights, which means that, overall, your baby will experience more hours of crying.

So, while I can't claim to know what your wee, two-month-old baby is thinking, my suspicion is that, if you're rocking him or patting his belly, he's trying to say something like this: "Hey! You dunderheads! Yes, you! The people right here! I know you're here because I can feel you rubbing my belly. I want to BREASTFEED! Get it? Breastfeed! Is that so hard to understand? Why are you just standing there and rubbing my belly? I don't want a belly rub! I want my breastmilk! Give me my milkie right NOW, for darn tootin'!"

Or I could be wrong.

Really, I can't get into your child's head.

If you choose to go with the lots-of-soothing approach, maybe your baby is thinking: "Alrighty then. I am still super upset that you're not breastfeeding me, which is why I'm sobbing so hard, but your reassuring belly pats are for sure helping me feel totally *Zen* about this sleep-training business right now. Totally fine with it. Don't let my wailing make you think otherwise. Wah. Wah."

Put your plan in writing.

It helps to write down your night-weaning goal on a piece of paper, so when it's 3:45 am and you've already endured two hours of crying and you're seriously second-guessing whether night-weaning is a good idea, you can look at that piece paper and remind yourself that your plan is *only one nursing between bedtime and 4 am*. Full stop. End of story.

Tell a friend.

Sharing your night-weaning plans with your partner or a sleep consultant or a sympathetic friend will make you feel accountability for them, which will in turn make you keep working to reach your sleep goal. According to research, when you share a goal with a person you value, rather than simply keeping it to yourself, you are twice as likely to take action and stay motivated to get the outcome you desire. It's human nature to care what others think of us, so telling someone can help light a fire within you and create the mindset that you deserve to be well rested and happy and live your best life. So seek out a buddy. Seek a buddy who doesn't make you feel pressured and who makes you feel like they have your best interests in mind. A sympathetic friend, peer, spouse, or consultant can help you do this.

Brainstorm ideas for soothing *yourself*, Momma.

Have a game plan for how you're going to make it through the most uncomfortable bits of partial night-weaning. This is where the internet and your mom friends might have some good ideas. Surround yourself with support.

Be strong. And be prepared to stick it out for four or five nights.

New rule: Parents who abandon night-weaning or sleep-training after one or two or three nights aren't allowed to declare that they "tried sleep-training but it didn't work." You have to be willing to commit to four or five nights in a row, or it doesn't count. If you feel you only have it in you to tolerate three nights of crying, max, then maybe partial night-weaning is not for you. Why go through the difficult experience of allowing your baby to cry and cry if you pull the plug too early for it to lead to any change in the length of your baby's nighttime sleep?

Bear in mind that night-weaning isn't just an aspirational thing that only rare babies achieve. It really can be done once momma and daddy (more so than baby) are ready to stick with the process.

On the other hand, be flexible.

Night-weaning is more art than science. Use your judgment. If baby is still crying for several hours on Night 6, as the parent you need to make the call on whether to postpone partial night-weaning for another month or so. Your baby can't do it for you.

If you like, weigh your baby.

If it helps assuage your concerns, you can weigh your baby more frequently during this period. Babies typically gain 140 to 245 grams (4 2/3 to 8 ¾ oz) per week at this stage. If your baby's growth continues to be satisfactory to health professionals, then you can rest assured that he's still getting the nutrition he needs to thrive, even as he's sleeping for longer stretches at night.

Do use a clock.

When a baby is crying, two minutes can seem like 20 minutes and two hours can seem like five. Use a clock to keep track of the actual elapsed time.

I hope it's obvious that you should _not_ use a baby monitor.

Using a baby monitor to amplify the sound of sleep-training would be sheer torture.

Obviously you can hear your baby crying.
Without the monitor.

Remember, if you want to cut back on nursing at night, then the solution is to cut back on nursing at night.

Some people mistakenly advise mom to cut down on daytime nursing in order to achieve nighttime weaning. This is counter-productive. Cutting down on daytime nursing will just lead to less daytime nursing. It's too early to day-wean.

Of course it's okay to respond to your baby at night!

Once you've successfully night-weaned, *do* get up to nurse baby in the middle of the night if he asks for it. Just because you've gone through the process of night-weaning doesn't mean that you've now committed to ignoring your baby's cries every night from now until he moves out of the house.

After the night-weaning process is complete, your baby will have fewer wakings—but not *every* single night. If there's the odd night when he wakes up more often than the **one or zero** times that you were expecting him to nurse, it could be because he's going through a growth spurt or fighting off a cold or chilled because his blanket has slipped off.

Once they've caught up on sleep, mommas usually don't mind the occasional, extra-special night-nursing session.

It's normal to night-wean more than once.

The majority of moms who night-wean find they have to go through the night-weaning process at least one more time at some point. This sometimes happens after baby has been ill or working hard on a new tooth or enjoying a vacation—anything that throws off the usual routine. For example, maybe you were staying at a friend's house for a week and your eight-month-old baby started waking up because he was in a strange place, and you were night-nursing him to keep him from waking your hosts. Now you're back home and—voilà! You have a baby who's getting up twice *every* night again. Just know that this is normal and expected. You simply need to go through the night-weaning process again, once you're ready.

The good news is that night-weaning the second or third time around is usually *a lot shorter and easier* than it was the first time. Having to night-wean your child a second or third time is not a big deal.

Some so-called experts claim that this fact—the reality that at some point most night-weaned babies revert back to a regular night-waking habit and need to be night-weaned again—is proof that night-weaning isn't effective. To which I say: *Hello, did you miss the whole bit where momma finally got night after night of restorative sleep?*

Other self-proclaimed experts say this regression is proof that night-weaning isn't "natural," or not right, but that doesn't follow either. On vacation I happily revert to my 20-year-old self: late bedtimes, glorious sleep-ins, copious quantities of wine, and no care for who's doing the laundry or how we're managing to pay for groceries—but that doesn't mean the vacation version of me is more "natural" or better.

You can do it! You can take back the night!

It's time for mommas to push back against the unhelpful orthodoxy: *Never let a baby cry himself to sleep.* Says who? Using what evidence? Just because an endlessly reiterated statement is passed on with the ring of authority doesn't make it true. We need to take back the night, mommas! You and your baby deserve every minute of replenishing sleep you can get.

Give a good night's rest a try, and wonderful things will begin to happen. Just wait and see!

Speaking of taking back the night, figure out what you're doing for birth control.

If you're formula feeding, your first menstrual period usually comes six to eight weeks after your baby's birth.

If you're breastfeeding, your first menstrual period may begin six to eight weeks post-partum as well, but many breastfeeding mommas experience amenorrhea (no menstrual periods) for longer. Your period may not come back until weaning begins.

Pregnancy *can* occur before your first period, though, so you may want to discuss birth control options with a medical professional sooner rather than later.

CHAPTER 8:

Three Months Old

"Bliss was it that dawn to be alive
But to be young was very Heaven!"

– William Wordsworth, *The Prelude* (1799)

In the daytime, continue breastfeeding on demand.

When he's awake in the daytime, your growing baby continues to need frequent breastfeeding. Whenever he seems unsettled, offer him some of your sweet momma milk.

> **Good to know!**
>
> Expect 24 to 48 hours of increased feeding when baby has growth spurts at one, three, six weeks & at three months.

Watch for baby to move bedtime even earlier.

Back when your baby was a newborn, he was falling asleep for the night between 9 pm and midnight. Then, sometime after about 40 days, he naturally developed an earlier bedtime, likely between about 8 and 11 pm.

At three to four months of age, watch for another change: your baby showing drowsy signs and being ready for bed even earlier—likely between **6 and 8 pm**.

Follow his lead, because at this stage the earlier bedtime is a baby-led development. As soon as you see a lull in his activity, glazed-over eyes, or yawning, it's time to start the process of soothing your baby to sleep.

Firm up your baby's first morning nap.

For the first few months, babies can sleep anytime, anywhere during the day. But by five months of age, most babies settle into a fairly predictable napping schedule. This transition, from the Wild West of sleeping to a fairly predictable nap routine, takes place at a slightly different pace and at slightly different ages for each unique baby. These variables aside, **the order** in which the transitions occur is fairly consistent for all babies.

If transitioning to a predictable daytime napping routine is like a marathon, then consider an earlier night bedtime as the starting whistle. It's easiest to settle baby into a predictable, consolidated daytime-napping schedule when mom and dad begin working on it soon after baby has—on his own—moved his night bedtime to between 6 and 8 pm.

In other words: *After* baby has moved his night bedtime to between 6 and 8 pm, *then* mom and dad can begin working on transitioning the first morning nap from a random wherever/whenever flake-out to something that recurs on a timed schedule.

Generally, though, most babies are ready around now.

When they're around three months of age (or three months after their original due date for babies born early), most babies are highly amenable to a scheduled *first* morning nap.

There are two key guidelines to keep in mind when establishing a morning-nap schedule for a baby who's around 12–16 weeks old:

✓ The timing is based on elapsed time, not clock time.

✓ Crying is expected, but should be minimal.

Time the morning nap according to elapsed time.

Most 12- to 16-week-old babies get up for the day between 6 and 9 am. Once your three-month-old is up, write down his wake-up time on a sticky note. Then add 1 hour *and* add 1.5 hours.

Let's say baby woke up for the day at 7 am. On your paper, jot down 7, 8, and 8:30 am. This means that at 7 am you'll open the curtains, welcome bright sunlight into your home, and enjoy some lovely, active one-on-one time with your baby. Then, somewhere **between 8 and 8:30 am**, as soon as you see the slightest lull or slowing in your baby's movements, begin the soothing-to-sleep routine.

Because your three-month-old baby's scheduled nap is based on elapsed time, and not a pre-set time, it will occur at a different time every morning. The important part is to begin a soothing-to-sleep routine within 1 to 1.5 hours of morning wake-up time.

Crying may happen, but should be minimal.

Once you've nursed your three-month-old baby to sleep for his first morning nap (or as close to asleep as you can—babies don't always fall asleep at the breast, even if you want them to), **one of four scenarios** will occur:

- ✓ Scenario #1: Your baby, who fell asleep at your breast, stays asleep once you put him down and has a nap that lasts at least 20 minutes.
- ✓ Scenario #2: Your baby, who didn't quite fall asleep before unlatching from your breast, promptly passes out once you lay him in his bassinet, and stays asleep for at least 20 minutes.
- ✓ Scenario #3: Your baby, who managed to fall asleep at your breast, wakes up the moment you place him in his bassinet and he begins to cry; or, he wakes up and begins crying after less than 20 minutes of sleeping.
- ✓ Scenario #4: Your baby, who didn't quite fall asleep before unlatching from your breast, begins to cry the moment you place him in his bassinet.

With Scenarios #1 or #2, there's nothing further you need to keep track of once the initial twenty minutes are up. Just promptly go and pick up your baby as soon as he wakes up.

But with Scenarios #3 or #4, you'll need take a deep breath, because you now need to prepare for 20 solid minutes of hard-core parenting. Not just hard-core parenting. You need to do the *hardest* parenting.

Are you up for it?

Are you mom enough?

Can you deal?

Okay, here goes: For 20 whole, long, heartbreaking minutes you do…*nothing.*

Make sure you actually write down the two time periods on a piece of paper—from the minute you place baby (whether he is asleep or awake) in his bassinet to the minute when the 20 minutes are up—because if you don't, two elapsed minutes will feel like 10 and 20 elapsed minutes will feel like an hour.

Although maybe, on the other hand, if you already chose to do night weaning a few weeks ago, you might be feeling that 20 minutes is not such a big deal. During night-weaning, a momma might give her baby permission to cry for as much as two hours or so before he drifts back to sleep. When it comes to establishing a scheduled, daytime morning nap for a three-month-old, though, most mommas agree that it's best to limit the crying to about 20 minutes. You might find 20 minutes quite doable if you've already experienced night-weaning—and the relief that comes with seeing your baby wake up bubbly, gurgling, cooing and smiling the morning after a night-weaning session (and a good night's rest).

Once you've walked away from your crying baby, one of two subsequent scenarios will occur:

- ✓ Your baby cries very hard for what feels like an eternity, and then he cries softly for what feels like another interminably long period, and then—**after less than a total of 20 minutes of crying**—he falls asleep, *or*
- ✓ Your baby cries the entire 20 minutes.

Once the initial 20 minutes are up, if he's fallen asleep then you can let him keep sleeping until he wakes up—at which point promptly go get him.

On the other hand, once the 20 minutes are up, if he's still awake and crying, you have two options. You can either try to soothe baby to sleep again (if you get the sense he was quite close to falling asleep), or you can pick him up and try the scheduled morning nap again tomorrow—or next week, or the week after that. Some babies are more amenable to a scheduled morning nap at three months old and some are more amenable at four months old. As momma, you get to make the call, based on what you feel is best for your baby.

Also: Some babies won't cry at all when this first morning nap is being established, while other babies will. It's partly the luck of the draw and partly expert timing.

Ah, expert timing.

Expert timing can be elusive. It involves nailing that fleeting moment when baby is ideally primed to ride the sleep wave back into slumber—so not too early, when he's still in biological awake mode; and not too late, when he's overtired and wired. It also involves nailing the exact age when baby is ready to seamlessly transition to a scheduled morning nap—so not too early, when he's too young; and not too late, when mom and dad have inadvertently reinforced jack-in-the-box-morning-nap behaviour for longer than necessary.

Of course, if you don't pull off this ambitious expert timing, no worries. Few people can. It just means that instead of *no* tears you'll have *some* tears today, and that's okay.

It helps to keep in mind that any crying that occurs as you work on establishing this first morning nap isn't because you're doing something to *make* your baby cry. It's because you're *allowing* your baby to cry. If your baby is upset about his morning nap, let him share that feeling with you.

As a bonus, any self-soothing skills your child starts working on now—while riding that last crest of the sleep wave into slumber—will count towards the 10,000 hours of practice he needs to handle whatever frustrations life's going to throw at him. Whether it's another toddler—in a few months—walking off with a toy he wasn't done playing with, someone ghosting him on social media in adolescence, or a boss (a stupid, stupid boss) giving him a pink slip in adulthood, your baby will need to build up reserves for those moments when the going gets tough. Feeling upset and then recovering is how we develop resilience.

In English, we sometimes admonish upset people to "calm down," but I prefer the phrase in French: "*calme soi*"—calm *yourself*. Establishing a scheduled early-morning nap at three months of age will give your baby a bite-sized practice run at self-calming.

Soothe your baby without tears for the remainder of his naps.

After the timed first nap in the early morning, your three-month-old baby will continue to need naps throughout the rest of his day. For these additional naps, look to your baby for signs of drowsiness, rather than trying to time them according to a pre-set schedule. In general, though, babies at this age are ready for a nap after one to two hours of wakefulness. And they tend to save their longest period of wakefulness for the end of the day.

The key difference between the first morning nap and other daytime naps at this age is that there's no need to coach your baby into having the latter. If your baby falls asleep, then let him sleep. If he doesn't fall asleep, pick him up and carry on with your mom-and-baby adventures. **The first morning nap** is the only one where you allow your **three-month-old baby** to cry for **up to 20 minutes**.

Baby-proof your baby's immediate environment.

As soon as your baby learns to move his hands to his mouth, he'll want to put everything in it. Be on the lookout for small objects that can pose a hazard, especially batteries, marbles, buttons, coins, needles, safety pins, scissors, forks, knives, makeup, medicines, and household cleaners.

Now and then, have a heart-to-heart chat.

If you're looking for something fun to do together, nothing rivets young babies' attention more than mom or dad's face and voice. So every now and then, spend a few minutes looking at and goo-goo-talking to your baby.

Babies this age operate on a slow time scale. Researchers Alyson Shapiro and John M. Gottman analyzed interactions between parents and their three-month-olds and found that, if a father sticks his tongue out at his baby, the child might imitate him, but a minute or two later. This is because, for baby, the feat takes great effort. Only those parents who continue to focus on the present moment have the pleasure of witnessing their child's response.

Sometimes we can get wrapped up in the dry business of caring for baby: feeding, sleeping, changing diapers. On occasion, carve out some special time to really enjoy your delightful little bugaboo.

CHAPTER 9:

Months Four and Five

Baby is now ready for a more predictable sleep schedule.

Until recently, your baby could fall asleep anytime, anywhere, amidst any amount of noise. This, however, is about to change.

By the age of four months, your baby will prefer to nap in a quiet, darkened room, away from most household noise. This doesn't mean you need to maintain monastic silence. Once they've fallen asleep, infants typically stay asleep, even with doorbells ringing and fire alarms wailing. It just means you should no longer expect baby to doze off easily in a busy restaurant.

Another change is that, by the age of four months, your baby will sleep best in a bassinet, bed, or crib. *Newborn* babies are amenable to having both portable naps (in a stroller, swing, baby carrier, or while being held) and stationary naps (in a bassinet, bed, or crib). Anything goes. By the age of four months, however, your baby will have longer, more restorative sleeps if you cut out the portable naps. So, no more naps in a car, stroller, baby swing or carrier, or in momma's arms. The occasional exception is fine, of course, but mobile naps should no longer be your regular go-to.

To help you get the logic behind this, think back to the last time you fell asleep during a car ride. The minute the car stopped, you immediately woke up, right? That's what makes mobile sleeps inferior as your baby gets older. Past the newborn stage, it's hard for humans to get into a deep sleep on the move.

Another change: Many parents stop regularly swaddling somewhere between the ages of two and five months old. Swaddling is not recommended once baby can roll over, because the constriction poses a risk for suffocation.

Silence, stillness, and no more swaddling. Big changes. And that's not all. When it comes to sleep, a lot more is about to change....

Next step: Convince *yourself*, Momma, that baby is ready for a sleep schedule.

This is going to be a busy couple of months. There's a *lot* of sleep-training that goes on at this stage. So clear your calendar, cancel your coffee dates. We're sleep-training.

Just to clarify: Sleep-training is not the same thing as night-weaning, even though the two are often conflated.

Dr. Marc Weissbluth, a pediatrician and sleep researcher, coined the now-familiar phrase "sleep-training" to describe the practice of establishing a set, consolidated schedule for morning and afternoon naps, and an early evening bedtime.

While establishing a schedule may sound a tad regimented, caregivers have long known that predictable routines and rituals are comforting for small children. They help them learn what to expect from their environment and provide them with a reassuring sense of security: All is right with the world.

Babies are naturally ready for a predictable sleep schedule at this age.

Sleep-training happens now, and not at the newborn stage, because somewhat predictable bedtimes and longer sleep patterns naturally begin to emerge around the three- to four-month mark. For this reason, sleep-training is easiest (read: involves the least crying) when it is initiated (*initiated*—not necessarily completed) between about 12 and 16 weeks (or 12 to 16 weeks after the original due date for babies born early).

And, chances are, that's exactly what you did last month—you *initiated* sleep-training. Last month, you probably worked on establishing a scheduled first morning nap for your three-month-old baby.

Over the next couple of months, you'll work on finishing what you started by consolidating your baby's remaining daytime and nighttime slumber into three or four predictable sleep times.

While sleep-training is *easiest* at this age, I'm going to level with you: it's still hard. Babies are mysterious. They reach certain milestones on their own, without any intervention. Others require parents to roll up their sleeves and really get in there. This is one of those milestones that many babies resist.

Some claim that babies' resistance to a "parent-imposed" sleep schedule is proof that sleep-training is unnatural. But the fact remains: It works. Babies who are sleep-trained at around three to five months of age get better sleep. Babies who get better sleep are less fussy during their awake times, and less fussy during awake times means fewer tears overall.

Plus, it's not exactly a parent-imposed sleep schedule. There's a biological, neurological basis for sleep-training around three-to-five months of age—rather than at two months of age or at six months of age.

Adults enter into sleep with a non-REM period. After that, they cycle through phases throughout their slumber, from light, non-REM-sleep to deep, non-REM sleep to REM sleep (which is when we dream). Every 90 minutes or so, when cycling back to a light sleep stage, we all experience a partial awakening. Adults who don't suffer from insomnia aren't even aware of these light arousals throughout the night—they simply ride the sleep wave back into the next cycle of slumber.

Unlike adults, newborn babies enter directly into REM sleep. Just like that! No messing around with the non-REM sleep at the start of a snooze.

But then—around the age of three to four months—something changes and infants also begin to enter sleep with a non-REM period, just like adults. This makes them sensitive to light and noise and movement, which means they need a quiet, dark, non-mobile environment for deeper, more restful slumber.

As Dr. Weissbluth learned through his research and clinical practice, if mom and dad don't realize this change is coming—and so neglect to follow baby's biological rhythms and make adjustments to how and when they put baby to bed—then their child will become overtired. Once a person at any age becomes overtired, it becomes harder to fall asleep, stay asleep, and get a good rest.

In other words, establishing a 9 am morning nap, a 1 pm afternoon nap, and a 6:30 pm bedtime does not constitute forcefully regimenting a routine. If it were, then parents would have the freedom to impose anything they want: *Morning nap starting at 5 am! Afternoon nap starting at 3 pm! Bedtime at 4:30! Sleep-training for a set naptime schedule starting at six weeks!*

Instead of thinking of it as the adult imposing a routine, think of sleep-training the other way around: Parents start sleep-training when their baby is between three and five months of age in order to follow *baby's* body clock. You're not scheduling your baby—after all, the random napping he was doing until now gave you freedom and you were perfectly happy with it. Rather, your baby's biology is scheduling *you*. If anything, Momma, *you're* the one who should be crying here. How on earth are you going to head out to meet your new momma friends when you're trapped by a nap?

Most babies cry during sleep training and that's okay.

Sometime in the 1990s or early 2000s (I think around the time the Sears series of attachment-parenting books were being released and horror stories of Ceausescu-era Romanian orphanages were permeating the zeitgeist), the parenting pendulum began swinging towards an extreme: Never let your baby cry. Not ever. What makes this babycare book different from the babycare books of the past quarter-century or so is that I'm willing to say something out loud that the mommas who are part of the Last Analog, Millennial and Pandemonnial generations[30] have already been confiding to one another in conspiratorial whispers: *The game plan was to use **gentle** approaches to nudging baby to sleep, but in the end* (cue the downcast eyes, sideways glance, and hushed tone), *I just couldn't handle it anymore, and we let our baby cry.*

The word "gentle" is a red herring, a misleading clue. It's a claim that doth protest too much. There's a reason why the internet and babycare coaches and parenting books don't promise you "gentle" methods of changing diapers or breastfeeding or cuddling or counting your baby's pudgy little toes. It's because we already know we can do all of those things without making baby upset. The fact that every sleep consultant is now promising the holy grail of "gentle," when it comes to sleep, should be your first clue that maybe there's something not so gentle about the whole process. I'd love to see a sleep-training consultant promise parents an uncomfortable approach to sleep-training. That would be refreshingly honest.

What's normal for crying? How do I know when to intervene?

I mentioned this in an earlier chapter, but I'll repeat it here so you don't have to go flipping back through the pages. There aren't any rules of thumb for how much crying is too much crying during sleep-training, so you'll have to listen to your mom gut. The best I can do is pass on wisdom from other moms who've been there before you:

- If your baby carries on really intensely or powerfully for 15 or 20 minutes without stopping and then settles, that's fine.

---

30   Baby Boomers (born 1945-1965; reached adulthood 1965-1985)
     Generation X (born 1960-1980; reached adulthood 1980-2000)
     Humanity's Last Analog Childhood Generation (born between 1975 and 1995; reached adulthood between 1995 and 2015)
     Millennials (b. 1990-2010; reaching adulthood 2010-2030); and
     Pandemonnials (b. 2005-2025; reaching adulthood 2025-2045)

- If the cry is lower pitched than a panicked or pained crying, then you don't need to worry.

- If the tone says he's mad or sad, let him process those strong feelings. They're his feelings. He has a right to feel them. If you hear a cry that says, "I'm absolutely terrified," then you'll want to step in and save him.

- If the crying is really intense for five or ten minutes, and then there's a lull, after which baby gets worked up again, then stops again—in other words, if the crying comes in little peaks—and your baby does that for an hour or so, the moms who've been there before you say don't worry about it.

If sleep training is natural, then why is there crying involved?

Sometimes parents assume that the crying that occurs during the relatively brief sleep-training period—when a consistent schedule is being established—is an indication that their baby is uniquely unsuited to the routine of a morning nap, afternoon nap, and early bedtime. But the reality is that your four-month-old baby has a lot in common with almost every other four-month-old baby out there. Just as most adults feel a little drowsy after lunch, and again after 9 pm, babies at this age begin experiencing both a dip in body temperature and an increase in drowsiness at predictable times of the day.

So, if Mother Nature intended babies to establish regular sleep routines at this age, then why—oh *why*—is there crying involved?

I don't know.

I really don't know.

Perhaps one day some brilliant researcher will discover a neurological or evolutionary imperative behind the resistance to sleep scheduling. Personally I wonder if maybe our hunting and foraging ancestors had the whole tribe go down for a morning and afternoon siesta, which would have made it easier for a baby to nap, then, too. Maybe our babies are just still having a hard time adjusting to the Agricultural Revolution that took place 11,000 years ago, and then (fast forward a few thousand years) the invention of the lightbulb and the concept of scheduling lifestyles around the workweek and retail operating hours. Maybe the real enemy is modernity.

But that's for another day. Right now you have a four-to-five-month-old baby before you and that four-to-five-month-old baby is officially no longer suited to napping randomly wherever and whenever the mood strikes. He'll thrive with a nap schedule and setting this nap schedule *will* involve crying.

If your goal is to minimize unnecessary crying, there's an irony to consider. What ultimately motivates parents to sleep-train is the knowledge that their child will, overall, end up crying *less*, not *more*. There will be crying for only a few days while the nap schedule is being established; after that the vast majority of bedtimes begin tear-free. That sounds a lot less painful than chronic crying, wherein a cranky, sleep-deprived child suffers a meltdown during his body's biological spike in drowsiness every single morning, afternoon, and evening for the next two years.

In other words, you can think of a cry-it-out sleep-training method as the ultimate no-cry sleep solution. *Super*!

Okay, ready for sleep-training? Yes?

Come now…Stick with me…because, well, you've come this far with me already.

You can do this!

Start the sleep-scheduling process by establishing a 6:30 pm bedtime.

Until now your baby has been in charge of determining his night bedtime and this bedtime probably falls between 6 and 8 pm. If your baby's self-selected bedtime is falling closer to 8 pm or later, the first step in sleep-training is to help you convince your four- or five-month-old baby to move his bedtime as close to 6:30 pm as possible. If your baby's self-selected bedtime is already falling around or before 7 pm *(what a good baby!)*, then you can skip this section.

Here's how you start

Sometime after 6 pm, once your baby begins fussing, nurse him to sleep, or as close to asleep as you can (babies don't always fall asleep at the breast, even if you want them to). Sometimes moms are mistakenly advised to unlatch while baby is "drowsy but still awake" for sleep-training purposes, but this isn't necessary. Nursing your baby to sleep (if your baby is into falling asleep at the breast) will in no way interfere with establishing a 6:30 pm bedtime.

Once he's asleep—or at least drowsy, as the case may be—put him down in his bassinet or crib.

As soon as you do that, there's a decent possibility he'll start crying. After all, he wasn't planning on turning in for the night. He just wanted a bit of milko to keep him going, and then he was planning to stay up and watch Netflix with mom and dad.

Give it one full hour.

Here's the hard part: Say goodnight to your crying baby, step away, and leave the room.

Next, give your sobbing baby **one hour** to figure out how to ride the sleep wave back into slumber. Check the time. Let's say your kitchen clock says 6:40 pm. If your baby is crying and crying and crying, you'd wait until around 7:40 pm before going back to pick him up and soothe away his tears (typically with nursing).

If you ended up having to pick up your baby after an hour, that's okay. You now have two equally valid options.

One option is to try to nurse your baby to sleep again, and to then wait another hour. This may be the right choice if you sense your baby was very close to drifting off to sleep.

Another option is to leave the sleep-training behind for tonight and try again another night. You can just hang out together for a while and then nurse him to sleep, following your normal routine, at *his* self-selected later bedtime.

Either of these options will work: choose what you feel will work best for your family tonight.

Regardless of which option you choose, use your judgment to decide whether your baby is close to being ready for an earlier bedtime (in which case, try sleep-training again tomorrow) or if he's not yet ready (in which case, perhaps wait a week or so before trying again).

The finish line

You've nailed it when you can check both these two boxes:

- ❐ You nurse baby down to sleep for the night sometime around 6:30 pm and, once you put him in his bed, he ends up asleep after either no crying or less than two minutes of crying. **AND**

- ❐ He **stays asleep**.

"Stays asleep" means your baby sleeps for **one of the following** two chunks of time:

- ✓ **A baby who's been partially night-weaned.** Baby wakes up once or twice or not at all between bedtime and the morning wake-up.

- ✓ **A baby who is nursing on demand throughout the night.** Four- to five-month-old babies who haven't been partially night-weaned tend to wake up every couple of hours (when they naturally cycle into the light, non-REM stage of sleep) for some comfort nursing. Many moms who share a bed with baby say they hardly wake up during these brief, nighttime nursing sessions.

> **Here's a typical experience of establishing an earlier bedtime, shared by a mom of one:**
>
> - Night 1: baby cried for 1 hour. I then picked him up, and tried again to nurse him down to sleep. After putting him down the second time, he cried for 55 minutes and then fell asleep for the night.
> - Night 2: Cried for 45 minutes, then fell asleep for the night.
> - Nights 3, 4, and 5: 20 minutes of crying each night.
> - Nights 6, 7, 8, 9: 10 minutes of crying each night.
> - Night 10: Less than 60 seconds of crying.
> - Night 11: No crying. Baby fell asleep at my breast and stayed asleep when I put him down. This is now our new normal!

Next step: Convince your four- or five-month-old baby to have a predictable 9 am nap.

Sometime around four-to-five months of age, babies are ready to schedule all their daytime naps. Rather than sleeping at varying times of the day for varying lengths of time, babies at this age are ready to consolidate all of their daytime sleep into two or three relatively consistent naptimes.

To help with timing, wait until you've comfortably established a night bedtime around 6:30 or 7:00 pm before tackling daytime naps.

Once you and your baby are ready, we'll start by working on your baby's ability to fall asleep in his own crib for a morning nap. We don't want to tackle the afternoon nap quite yet. We're taking this sleep-training one bedtime at a time.

Didn't we already establish the morning nap?

We sure did! If you were able to establish a morning nap when your baby was around three months old, then you can skip this section. Done and done!

The main difference between establishing the morning nap at three months of age versus at four or five months of age is that when baby is three months old, families generally limit any nap-training crying to 20 minutes. Whereas if baby is working on this milestone at four or five months of age, some families have to let baby cry for as long as an hour to establish the morning nap.

Monotony warning

Writing instructors say: Never bore your reader. And yet, my test readers have told me this section is a tad humdrum. So what to do? Liven it up with enthralling anecdotes? Thought-provoking metaphors? A cameo from a celebrity? (Harry Styles says "Hi!")

There's no getting around it. A step-by-step breakdown of how to sleep-train makes for monotonous reading.

On the other hand, my testers have said that the step-by-step sequence in this chapter is helpful, and it works. So I'm going to go out on a limb here and just keep the boring bits. If you feel your eyes glazing over, I'm so, so sorry, but try to stick with me. It's worth it.

All right, let's do this. Who's pumped? I'm pumped! Let's establish a 9:00 am nap!

Everyone starts off with the same first six steps.

If you haven't yet established the morning nap, here are the first six steps to follow for a baby who is four months old or older:

1. Once your baby has been up for one to two hours and you notice a hint of slowing or fussing in his movements (let's say, for our example, at about 8:30 am or so), nurse him to a state of drowsiness. There's a good chance he'll fall asleep at your breast, but it's okay if that doesn't happen. As long as baby is in a drowsy state, you've done a good enough job.
2. Put baby down in his crib.
3. Leave.

4. Write down the time. For example, <u>let's say it's 9:20 am</u> when you come down from his bedroom.
5. At this point, most babies begin to cry. And cry and cry.
6. Wait at least 60 minutes (10:20 am in this example).

Your baby's crying is very difficult to listen to, so I want to give you a big hug and reassure you that it will get better. The first time takes the longest, but it's worth it when your resolve outlasts your baby's persistence.

Your subsequent steps depend on what happens next.

A few different scenarios may occur. Below I list four examples.

Scenario #1: Baby cries the full 60 minutes.

If this is your scenario, then your remaining steps are:

7. Once the 60 minutes are up, go in, pick him up and soothe his tears away. Nursing is a great way to calm him down. Sleep-training is now over for the day.
8. For his remaining daytime naps today, let him sleep anywhere, at any time, for any length of time, with no tears. Just remember to be on the lookout for drowsy signs within one to two hours of wakefulness.
9. On another day, try again to establish a 9 am morning nap. Use your judgment to decide *when* you should try again. If your baby is closer to five months old you might feel you should try again tomorrow. If your baby is closer to 16 weeks old, you might make the call to wait another week before trying again.

Scenario #2: Baby cries for a while, and then falls asleep for <u>less than 20 minutes</u>, and then wakes up crying again before the original 60 minutes are up.

If this is your scenario then your remaining steps are:

7. When you no longer hear baby crying, write down the time. There's no need to check on him—if you can't hear him crying, assume he's asleep.

8. At this age, if baby has been quiet for <u>less than</u> 20 minutes before he starts crying again, then it's too early to pick him up. For example, let's say you wrote down that he stopped crying at 9:30 am, but now he's started crying again at 9:40 am. This means you would leave him in his crib until about 10:20 am, which you originally set as your "leave baby for at least 60 minutes" point (remember, in the example I'm using, you left the room at 9:20 am).

9. Once the original 60 minutes are up, go in and soothe him. Sleep-training is now over for the day.

10. For his remaining daytime naps today, go with the flow and let him sleep anywhere, at any time, for any length of time, with no tears.

11. The fact that he briefly fell asleep during the 60-minute period is a positive sign. Consider trying again tomorrow to establish a 9 am morning nap.

Scenario #3: Baby cries for a while, and then falls asleep for <u>at least 20 minutes</u>, and then wakes up crying again before the original 60 minutes are up.

If this is your scenario then your remaining steps are:

7. Once you no longer hear baby crying, write down the time. You can assume he has fallen asleep.

8. If baby has been quiet for at least 20 minutes and then he wakes up and begins to cry again, go in and pick him up immediately, even if 60 minutes have not yet passed since you first put him down. For example, let's say your baby stopped crying at 9:30 am and then you hear him start crying again at around 9:50 am. It hasn't been a full hour since you first put him down at 9:20

am, but after 20 minutes of napping, your baby has done well enough for today. You can go in and pick him up. Sleep-training is now over for the day.

9. For his remaining daytime naps today, let him sleep anywhere, at any time and for any length of time, with no crying.

10. The fact that he fell asleep for at least 20 minutes during the 60-minute period is an excellent sign. Try again tomorrow to establish the 9 am morning nap.

Scenario #4: Baby cries for a while, then finally falls asleep, and is still sleeping when the original 60-minute mark passes.

If this is your scenario then your remaining steps are:

7. Once you no longer hear baby crying, write down the time. You can assume he's asleep.

8. <u>After an hour has passed</u> from when you *first* put him down (remember, that was 9:20 am in our example), you can pick him up as soon as he wakes up, <u>regardless of how long he has slept</u>. So, for example, let's say he stops crying at 10:15 am, after 55 minutes of crying. Even if you hear him crying at around 10:20 am, after just five minutes of quiet, go in and pick him up and soothe his tears away. Sleep-training is now over for the day.

9. For his remaining daytime naps today, do what you've been doing in the past. In other words, go with the flow for the rest of the day, and let him sleep anywhere, at any time and for any length of time, with no crying to sleep.

10. The fact that he briefly fell asleep during the 60-minute period is a positive sign. Consider trying again tomorrow to establish the 9 am morning nap.

Many parents find this process takes a couple of weeks.

It can take a couple of weeks, but some babies establish the morning nap much sooner. A well-rested baby can figure it all out in as little as three days.

You'll know you've achieved this particular milestone of sleep-training when you can check *ALL* the following boxes:

- ❒ You nurse baby down to sleep around 9:00 am[31] and he falls asleep after no crying or less than two minutes of crying.
- ❒ He stays asleep for at least 20 minutes.
- ❒ When he wakes up, he cheerfully babbles and coos to let you know he's up and it's time for you get him.

In other words, your baby will not cry during either the falling-asleep or wake-up parts of the 9 am nap. Once there are no more tears at either end of the morning nap, then you can consider this step done—you've now convinced your baby to go down for a 9 am nap!

Well done!

Lengthen that morning nap to at least 60 minutes.

So you now officially have a baby who's willing to fall asleep for a morning nap.

The next step is to help him gain the skills to stay asleep for at least 60 minutes.

You can work on this step and the next step concurrently. In other words, you can work on **lengthening baby's morning nap** at the same time that you slowly begin **to establish baby's afternoon nap**.

---

31 Whenever a specific time is listed for a bedtime in any section of this book, be flexible in applying it to your own family. At your house the actual time may vary by as much as 30 to 60 minutes, in either direction. After all, if I were to generalize that adults go to bed at 11 pm, there's a strong chance that in your particular case I might be off by an hour or so. When you're establishing (and later maintaining) a bedtime schedule, read your child's drowsy signs—not just the clock.

Some babies figure out on their own how to nap for at least an hour. If this is the case with yours, you can skip this step and move on to the next one.

Many babies, however, start out with a 9 am nap that lasts only around 20 minutes. If it took a bit of crying to get to this point, I know you're not going to want any more tears. But your growing baby has a physiological need for at least 60 minutes of sleep for his morning nap, so you're doing him a favour by trying to lengthen it.

Here's how you get started.

First, write down the time your baby falls asleep. Let's say your kitchen clock says 9:30 am after you put him down. Jot down the 9:30 am start and the 10:30 am end. Seeing these times in writing will help remind you that the plan is to leave your baby in his room until at least 10:30 am, when the 60-minute mark has passed.

In this example, let's say you hear your baby wake up and begin to babble happily around 9:50 am, after just 20 minutes of sleeping. What you do is this: leave him in his crib. After a while, let's say around 10 am, his babbling will become more insistent. It's hard, I know, but give him the space he needs to work on lengthening this nap. Around 10:10 am, perhaps you begin to hear fussing. At 10:20 am it's full-on bawling. You keep your eye on that clock, and, hard as it is, don't go in and get him until around 10:30 am.

After the initial 60 minutes are up (again, 10:30 am in this example), you can immediately go get baby and soothe away his tears. (Of course, if he's fallen asleep again and is still asleep at the 10:30 am mark, then you can wait until he wakes up before going to get him.)

This process may take a couple of weeks—although some babies lengthen their morning nap to a full hour after just a few days.

You'll know you've achieved this milestone when you can check ALL the following boxes:

❐ You nurse baby down to sleep around 9 am and he falls asleep after either no crying or less than two minutes of crying.

❐ He stays asleep for at least 60 minutes.

❒ When he wakes up, he cheerfully babbles and coos to let you know he's up, so you can come get him.

Once there are no more tears at either the fall-asleep or wake-up ends of the morning nap AND your baby is getting at least 60 minutes of sleep, then you can consider this step done! You did it! Good job!

This is the point at which many families begin using a baby monitor. If your baby is sleeping in another part of the house while you go about your day, a monitor will amplify your baby's cheerful wake-up babble so you can hear it as soon as it starts. Once you hear his rousing murmurs, you'll know it's time to promptly go and get baby from his crib. <u>Babies feel more secure when they know they can rely on a caring adult to come fetch them soon after they enter their **post-nap awake mode**—*before* they start crying.</u>

Keep working on that sleep schedule: Establish the 1 pm nap.

Oy, more crying.

But I think you know the drill now.

Babies are ready for a scheduled afternoon nap sometime after their morning nap is established. Some are ready for afternoon-nap training as early four-and-a-half months of age, while others need a few more weeks. The key is to wait until you're getting comfortable with the scheduled morning nap before tackling the afternoon nap.

The process for establishing the afternoon nap at this age is exactly the same as the one for establishing the morning nap for a four- or five-month-old. As soon you notice your baby begin to fuss, sometime after 11:30 am, and as long as it's been at least one hour since his last sleep, you can begin taking the same steps you followed for establishing the morning nap. (If you skipped over the section on establishing the morning nap because your baby had already started going down for a scheduled morning nap when he was three months old, then go have a look at it now. Nap training for a three-month-old baby versus for a four-to-five-month-old baby involves a slightly different approach, and you'll want to use the approach that works for four-to-five-month-old babies.)

As with the morning nap, babies tend to wake up after about 20 minutes at first. Again, you can stretch out that initial 20-minute afternoon nap by giving baby time to settle back down into another, deeper round of sleep.

You'll know you've achieved this milestone when you can check ALL the following boxes:

- ❐ You nurse baby down to sleep sometime between about 12 noon and 1 pm and he falls asleep in his crib after either no crying or less than two minutes of crying.
- ❐ He stays asleep for at least 60 minutes.
- ❐ When he wakes up, he cheerfully babbles and coos to let you know he's up and it's time for you to come get him.

Well done, Momma! You did it!

Go with the flow if there's a third nap.

Some babies have a third nap at this age and some don't.

The good news is that the third nap involves none of this nasty sleep-training and crying. It just happens organically. And there's no minimum length for this third nap.

The other lovely aspect of the third nap is that it's easy to let it happen wherever you want—either in the baby carrier or in arms or on a separate sleep surface (such as a crib or bassinet). A mobile nap is just fine for the third nap. Don't worry about keeping the house quiet, either. The third nap is casual.

If there is a third nap, just go with the flow. Also go with the flow if there isn't one. The third nap is very much like a newborn nap.

Making the soothing-to-sleep routine efficient

Your next task, once you've established the 9 am(ish) morning nap, the 12 noon(ish) afternoon nap, and the 6:30 pm(ish) night bedtime, is to make your sleep routine as brief as possible. Lingering over an hour-long bedtime routine is fine if you know you'll have that kind of spare time at your disposal every night for the next several years, but if you suspect you might not, then aim for a routine that's closer to 15 or 20 minutes.

Yet again, this is an example where two mutually exclusive rules can simultaneously be true in a non-parallel universe: Feel free to nurse baby down to sleep, but don't feel you need to keep nursing until he falls asleep.

If your four-month or older baby falls asleep at the breast within about 20 minutes, you're good. Nursing to sleep is just fine. But if your four-month or older baby is drowsy but still awake after about 20 minutes, you don't need to keep nursing until he's fully asleep.

And just to be clear: I'm talking about a baby who is well past the newborn stage at this point, and I'm also only talking about the nursing associated with the bedtime routine. If you're nursing your baby at any other time of the day or night, there's no need to limit yourself to 20 minutes. Nurse as long as you like. It's the nursing associated with a scheduled sleep time that's best kept short and sweet at this stage.

If you've nursed your sleep-trained baby for what seems like a reasonable length of time for a bedtime routine, and he starts to cry the minute you put him down in his crib, then you need to keep walking. Running back and forth to resume nursing will prolong the bedtime routine to the point where you'll become one of those exhausted mothers who claims, "My baby will only fall asleep if I crawl into bed with him for an hour and wait until he's deep into the REM phase before I extricate myself, ninja-like, by somersaulting silently across the carpet and out of the room."

All babies prefer to keep mom or dad right by their side until they're deep into the REM stage of sleep. One of the skills your baby is working on during the sleep-training period is how to slip into a deep and inky sleep on his own once the soothing process is done.

Have faith in your little bugaboo, Momma. He can do it!

Now for the easy part: Load the dishwasher.

While newborn babies will blissfully snooze in a loud restaurant, after the age of about four months, children sleep best in a quiet environment, with one notable exception: babies, toddlers, preschoolers and, really, children of all ages, find it easier to fall asleep at night if they can hear a dim, distant clatter of household noise.

For baby, the din of the dinner dishes being cleared, the dishwasher being loaded, tomorrow's lunches being prepared — these are the soothing sounds of nightly ritual. The night kitchen's familiar clatter is like a security blanket. It signals to your child that no matter what happened today, all is now right with the world. Tonight is just like last night, mom and dad are nearby, and it's safe to sleep.

Make it part of mom or dad's routine to leave kitchen chores for the brief period that comes immediately after you've kissed baby good night and stepped out of the bedroom.

Offer solid food around the age of five-and-a-half months.

That was a lot of information about baby sleep.

Switching gears, I'm going close this chapter with some information about feeding baby at this stage.

You don't have to wait until baby is six months old to offer solids.

If your baby is capable of sitting with little help (i.e., safely in a high chair or on your lap with minimal support), then you can begin offering him finger food.

I suspect that the old recommendation, to delay solids until six months of age, came about because of the challenges associated with exclusive spoon-feeding.

Spoon-feeding is a recent invention. It only began to replace baby-led feeding sometime in the 20th century.

With spoon-feeding, parents have full control of consumption. Back in the 20th century, this meant that babies who weren't yet ready for solids were forced to ingest Pablum. When a five-month-old baby who's not yet ready for solids is spoon-fed, he'll use his tongue to thrust the food out, but it's very easy for parents to override the tongue-thrust reflex and force the spoon into baby's mouth. The solution for forced spoon-feeding at ever-younger ages? Doctors eventually established a "wait-until-baby-is-six-months-old" convention. After doctors began recommending no solids before the age of six months, babies were less likely to have solid foods forced upon them before they were ready, because by six months of age the vast majority of babies have grown out of the tongue-thrust stage.

More recently, however, medical professionals have recognized that many infants show solid-food readiness a few weeks before they hit the six-month mark. In January 2019, the Canadian Paediatric Society released new guidance clarifying that solid foods should be introduced at "around six months of age" but "not before four months of age," and that the practice should be "guided by the infant's developmental readiness for food."[32] In other words, if you're allowing your baby to take the lead on feeding himself, you can start offering him solids as soon as he's old enough to sit upright with minimal support.

When parents provide their five-month-old baby with the opportunity to feed himself with his hands, they effectively eliminate the risk of feeding him too early, because he's taking the lead. If he does manage to get the food you've placed before him into his mouth and ingest it, then he's ready; if he doesn't, then he's not ready and there's no foul because no one has forced food into his mouth.

If you're allowing your baby to take the lead on feeding himself, you can start offering him solids as soon as he's old enough to sit at the table with the family for meals.

---

32 "Timing of introduction of allergenic solids for infants at high risk," Canadian Paediatric Society, Posted: January 24, 2019, cps.ca/en/documents/position/allergenic-solids

When offering food at five months, use the "rule of thumb."

Offer your baby chunks of food that are at least the size and shape of an adult thumb. His hands don't yet have the fine motor skills to grab anything much smaller than that. It'll be a few more months before he develops the pincer skills in his fingertips to pick up tiny Cheerios.

To start, put larger chunks of food within reaching distance and see what he does with them.

You can put the food directly on the tray or table in front of him. If you use a plate, he's likely to pick it up and fling it as part of his normal, age-appropriate exploration. So instead of adding the complication of a plate or bowl, keep things simple by "removing the middleman" and putting his food directly on the tray of his high chair.

Once you set larger chunks of food in front of baby, he'll reach for them—but can he get them? And if he gets them, can he pick them up? If he picks them up, can he aim them at his mouth? If he aims them at his mouth, is he coordinated enough to clamp down on the food, and then keep his tongue from pushing it back out again? And then chew? And then swallow?

As you can see, there are many skills involved in consuming food. There's no need to rush baby through them. But there's no reason to hold him back either. Around five-and-a-half-months, put food within his reach. Then let him experiment—without any expectations around whether he'll take anything in.

Your baby has some pretty powerful gums.

Some parents worry whether baby will be able to handle solid food right off the bat. Rice-cereal advertising is so ubiquitous that it's become ingrained in us that store-bought, spoon-fed mush should be baby's first food. Because it involves extra work on mom's part, even worse is the expectation that baby's first food should be *home-made*, organic, spoon-fed mush. Mush isn't necessary, regardless of whether it's store-bought or home-made, so save yourself the trouble and go directly to solid foods that are actually *solid*. You can make it soft, sure. Soft, but *solid*.

Even without teeth, your baby can do a decent job of mashing up the food in his mouth.

Even as you begin to introduce solids, continue breastfeeding on demand.

During awake times in the day, your growing baby continues to need frequent breastfeeding. Nurse him as often as he wants.

Speaking of which, starting solids is like starting breastfeeding.

There are parallels between the first breastfeeding and the first solid-food feeding. One is that very few people figure it out on Day 1. Both also involve, initially, a lot of awkward attempts without much success.

Another parallel between the early days of breastfeeding and the early days of solid-food feeding: it's messy, so it helps if baby is naked. If he's seated at the table in nothing but a diaper, you won't end up with tomato stains on his best onesie.

Gagging, coughing, and choking

When baby is in charge of what goes into his mouth, he has better control over how much of it actually makes its way down his throat. That being said, it helps if you're aware that babies who feed themselves do making gagging and coughing noises quite frequently. This is because Mother Nature conveniently placed the gag reflex very high up in a baby's esophagus to protect him from the possibility of food going down the wrong pipe. If baby starts hacking and gagging while feeding himself solids, your best bet is to sit back and let him work it out. No need for you to leap into immediate action—which might actually make things worse.

This is also why it's important to give your baby *large* chunks of food to feed himself with. It's possible to accidentally aspirate a teeny tiny morsel, but much more difficult to accidentally aspirate a thumb-sized piece of food.

Suggestions for early foods

Here are some large foods your baby can experiment with for his first few meals:

- ✓ A thumb-length piece of hamburger (babies need dietary iron in their meals starting around the age of five or six months). (But not a thumb-length wiener or hot dog – their smooth edges make them a choking hazard for babies.)
- ✓ A thumb-length piece of whatever other meat you've cooked for the family that evening.
- ✓ A thumb-length piece of roasted or cooked potato, broccoli, carrot, or other vegetable.
- ✓ A thumb-length piece of hamburger bun or other bread (preferably whole wheat).
- ✓ A semi-circle of frozen, whole-wheat pita bread. To avoid waste, stick a bag of pita in the freezer immediately after bringing it home, and then dole it out, still frozen, in semi-circle halves. A teething baby will find the frozen pita soothing on his gums.
- ✓ Half a banana.

This is a great age to focus on quality over quantity. There's no minimum requirement for how much your baby needs to consume, and he's not yet tugging on your sleeve and declaring "I'm huuungry!," so you're free to offer him only the good stuff.

Don't worry about variety, either, because at this stage your baby is likely to waste most of the food you give him anyway. Right now you're just offering him food to see what he does with it.

As the saying goes, "Under one, just for fun!"

Bon appetit!

CHAPTER 10:

Six Months Old

"What a strange machine man is! You fill him with bread, wine, fish, and radishes, and out comes sighs, laughter, and dreams."

—Nikos Kazantzakis, poet and novelist (1883–1957)

Begin offering a greater variety of solid foods.

Give your baby finger food.

If you haven't introduced solid foods already, then you definitely need to begin when your baby is six months old. If you delay the introduction of solid food much longer, you'll increase your baby's risk for developing food allergies, and you may also miss the critical window when he's most amenable to this big change in his diet.

So if you haven't yet done so, put some solid food in front of baby and see what he does. Babies who aren't ready for solids may play with the food, they might even taste it, but they won't get serious about eating it. Rest assured the day will come when that food makes it down the hatch.

Be cautious with certain textures.

Although it's normal for a baby to gag and spit out food while developing his chewing and swallowing skills, avoid (or modify) foods that are choking hazards until your child is between three and four years old. Foods that may cause problems include:[33]

- **Round or smooth foods like grapes, cherries, or hard candies.** To make rounded fruits and vegetables safe, cut them into four parts and take out the pits or seeds. Avoid hard candies until your child is about four years old.
- **Smooth, rounded foods like wieners or hot dogs.** To make them safe, cut into bite-sized pieces.
- **Hard foods like raw vegetables.** To make them safe, cook or steam to soften them, or grate them into small pieces.
- **Foods that stick to the roof of the mouth, like cream cheese or peanut butter.** For safety, spread cream cheese or peanut butter thinly.

***After* baby starts successfully feeding himself finger foods, *then* offer spoon-feeding.**

Once you know your baby's willing and able to feed himself, you can add spoon-feeding to his diet.

The best way to approach spoon-feeding is to have a look at the meal that the rest of your family is eating and figure out which part you can adapt to a spoon-feeding format.

Usually it's as simple as taking a fork to mush down food that's already soft because it's been baked or cooked.

Alternatively, you can stick half a cup of various bits of your meal into a blender or food processor. You can, for example, create a single mélange of the pot roast, yam fries, and steamed edamame beans you

---

[33] More examples are available here: cdc.gov/nutrition/InfantandToddlerNutrition/foods-and-drinks/choking-hazards.html

prepared for tonight, or blend up part of the fresh poké bowls you ordered in.

Once you've made your mush, use a baby spoon to serve tiny bits of it to your baby. Try touching the spoon to his mouth or cheek, signalling him almost the way you would with your breast. He'll open his mouth if he's interested or turn his head away if he isn't.

And a sour face doesn't necessarily mean he doesn't like it. It just means the taste surprises him!

Your baby will signal that his meal is over when he starts finger-painting with or spitting out his food, closing his mouth, turning his head away, vocalizing, or waving his hands in front of his mouth. When food flung exceeds food swallowed, he's done!

Once baby figures out how to consume finger foods and spoon-fed foods, offer <u>one</u> or <u>two</u> meals every day.

And don't worry about *how much* food your baby is eating. As long as medical professionals are happy with your baby's weight gain, there's no need to monitor how much food he consumes. Put food in front of him, but pay no attention to whether he eats it, or, if he does, how much. Respecting his hunger and satiety cues will contribute to healthy eating habits and reduce his lifetime risk of obesity

Include foods rich in iron and vitamin C.

Keep things simple: there's no need to buy food specially made for a baby. Your child can eat (or not eat) whatever the rest of the family is being served.

Be on the lookout, though, for foods rich in iron and vitamin C. Babies need those elements in their diet starting around halfway through their first year because the iron stored in their bodies at birth gets used up by the time they're six months old. Babies need iron for growth and development, which is why it's important to include iron-rich foods in baby's solids. Good sources of iron include strips of meat, cooked eggs, beans, and lentils. Babies also need foods that contain vitamin C, which helps their bodies absorb the iron in food.

Good sources of vitamin C include sweet potatoes, green beans, squash, broccoli, strawberries, oranges, mandarins, and mangoes.

Be sure that you *do* introduce potential allergens such as peanuts, fish, or eggs right off the bat.

If you wait too long, you increase baby's risk of developing food allergies.

> **Did you know?**
>
> The two biggest factors in increasing allergy risk are: (1) the presence of eczema; and (2) waiting too long to introduce potentially allergenic foods.

There was a nearly two-decade period when parents were given the opposite advice. In 2000, the American Academy of Pediatrics published a since-discredited recommendation that children at high risk of allergies avoid eggs until the age of two and peanuts and fish until the age of three. In the ensuing years, allergies to tree nuts, peanuts, eggs, and seafood skyrocketed. The American Academy reversed course in 2008, and the Canadian Paediatric Society followed suit in 2019. Current guidance actively encourages parents to start feeding children common allergy-causing foods as soon as they're ready to eat solids.[34]

There was also a time when parents were told to wait three days between introducing each new food, but this practice isn't necessary either. If you're feeding your baby food right from the family dinner table, each dish will be made of multiple ingredients anyway. It's probably impossible to separate them.

If you're worried that food or breastmilk are causing issues with your child (sleep challenges, crying, rashes, redness, bloating, stomach cramps, fatigue), go with the axiom "innocent until proven guilty." True food allergies are an immune-system response (think anaphylactic reaction), and they're relatively rare. Food intolerances—also called

---

[34] Source: "Timing of introduction of allergenic solids for infants at high risk," Canadian Paediatric Society, Posted: January 24, 2019, cps.ca/en/documents/position/allergenic-solids

"food sensitivities"—are a dime a dozen and shouldn't be considered an adverse reaction to food. If you suspect your child has an actual allergy (and not just a sensitivity), the gold standard is an oral food challenge—where a person eats a small amount of the suspected allergen under medical supervision. Restricting your child's diet without a *bona fide* medical diagnosis can lead to unnecessary nutrient deficiencies and contribute to an unhealthy relationship with food.

There's just one food that experts recommend delaying: honey, which is best introduced after baby is 12 months old due to the risk of botulism. Foods that can cause choking also aren't recommended until three years of age, unless they're modified so that they can't easily get lodged in baby's throat (e.g., cooked until soft, mashed, ground, etc.).

Pretty much everything else is fair game.

As the amount of solid food he consumes increases, the amount of mother's milk he ingests decreases.

Baby's intake of mother's milk will decrease as soon as he begins eating solid foods. This is a normal stage of breastfeeding; one that ideally happens with your baby controlling the overall amount of food and breastmilk he consumes.

Continue nursing on demand.

While milk production decreases as soon as baby starts solids, there's no need to do any active weaning when baby is six months old. Carry on with nursing on demand throughout the daytime. At this stage, your baby—who may have by now, on his own, reduced his nursing sessions to as few as five or six per 24-hour period—continues to get key nutrients from breastmilk, and he's not yet ready to wean fully.

Many moms find that nursing sessions typically take under 20 minutes at this stage. This may be where the mistaken advice to nurse newborn babies for 20 minutes per side came from—newborns aren't that efficient, but a six-month-old baby is likely to be.

Keep in mind, however, that on any given day the length and number of nursing sessions could increase if baby is dealing with sickness, hot weather, a missed nap, or some other calamity—so continue to let him be the final arbiter of how often and how long he breastfeeds. And all bets are off in the evening, when your baby may feel like venting the frustrations of a tough day by bobbing on and off the breast.

Sleep-training does contribute somewhat to the more predictable nursing pattern most babies develop by this age. By the time a sleep-trained baby is around five-and-a-half or six months old, his nursing patterns might look something like this (all times are approximate):

- Around 5 am, nurse back to sleep.

- Nurse somewhere between 7 and 8 am, when he wakes up from his night sleep.

- Somewhere between 9 and 10 am—nurse down for a morning nap.

- Around 11 am—maybe nurse after waking up from the morning nap.

- Somewhere between about noon and 2 pm—nurse down for an afternoon nap.

- Around 2 pm—maybe nurse after waking up from the afternoon nap.

- Between about 3 and 6 pm—although babies are past the worst of the evening fussies by this age, some still go back for frequent, short nursings in the late afternoon/early evening. Baby might also squeeze in a short third nap (perhaps between 3 and 5 pm) in-between these late-afternoon nursings.

- Around 6:30 pm—nurse down to sleep.

- Some six-month-old babies will then sleep through until morning, if mom and dad have chosen to do partial night-weaning, while others will wake up to nurse a few times throughout the night.

Again, though, please take all of the sample feeding/sleeping schedules in this book with a grain of salt. Just as you would if I said your adult schedule looks like this:

- 6:30 am wake-up.
- 7 am breakfast.
- 9 am bowel movement.
- 11:30 am lunch.
- 3 pm crash and burn—you're having trouble keeping your eyes open at your desk.
- 5:30 pm, arrive home and argue with spouse (we never truly outgrow our "evening fussies" period).
- 6 pm dinner.
- 11 pm fall asleep.

Your schedule probably doesn't look *exactly* like this. Especially not on the weekend (cue the nachos at 10 pm on Friday at the pub). But there may be some elements you recognize. It's the same with your baby. He won't follow the *exact* schedules I list throughout this book, but something pretty close.

And keep this in mind: Some babies are very predictable by five months of age, while others have irregular nursing patterns throughout the first year. *Both* scenarios are within the range of normal.

Keep soothing your baby down for his naps.

Bedtimes tend to be tear-free at this stage. Most days you'll lovingly nurse your baby down to sleep and he'll wake up calm and smiling. During awake times, you then have the satisfaction of hanging out with a happy, alert, well-rested, and easygoing baby.

Now that baby's naps are firmly established, you can give yourself a little flexibility with adhering to his sleep schedule. If you need to be out and about with baby during a nap or over the evening bedtime, it's fine to make the occasional exception. Just be aware that baby will likely nurse more often when you skip a nap or put him to bed late. This is because he knows he's not comfortable, but he doesn't quite know why. In a desperate attempt to make things right, he'll keep bobbing on and off the breast, hoping that some milkie will satisfy his need, which it won't, because what he really wants is sleep. Still, a mom who's open to nursing her overtired baby more frequently can buy some peace when he misses a nap because of a family excursion.

And while you can now make exceptions to his sleep schedule, be wary about skipping too many naps in a row. We're all born with a chronotype encoded in our DNA that determines our individual circadian rhythm: when we feel sleepy and when we feel alert. But lifestyle also plays a role in shaping our circadian rhythms. Adults with an erratic sleep schedule have a harder time falling asleep and staying asleep. The same holds true for babies who are older than four months. Be relatively consistent with your baby's sleep schedule at this stage and you'll be rewarded with a baby who sleeps like, well… a baby!

Schedule a visit with a health professional.

While there are many well-baby checkups in the earliest months, it may have been a while since your baby last visited a health professional.

By six months your baby should turn towards your voice and make babbling noises. If he isn't hitting these two milestones, be sure to let your doctor know. A hearing exam may be in order.

Earlier is also better when it comes to making sure your baby can see. A doctor likely checked your newborn's eyes, but around six months of age he's due for another eye check.

During your well-baby visit, you can also ask your physician what frequency she recommends for future checkups.

Baby-proof more parts of your house.

Your baby will become mobile very soon, so this is a good time to baby-proof your home. Don't wait until after you've spent five minutes—five very long, heart-pounding minutes—looking for the baby you last saw in your living room before realizing that today is the day he figured out how to crawl up the stairs all the way to the second floor, on his own.

When they start coming, certain developmental milestones arrive fast. It's not a case of: Go up one step, then sit there and bask in the glory. It's a case of: *All the way up!*

At your next well-baby visit, ask your health professional for information about baby-proofing. Some ideas to start you off:

- ✓ Avoid tablecloths.
- ✓ Keep breakable objects out of reach.
- ✓ Cover electrical outlets with safety caps.
- ✓ Keep hot liquids out of reach. Tea and coffee often cause burns for babies and toddlers. Also, when you're cooking, use the stove's back burners when you can; if you use the front burners, turn the pot handles toward the rear of the stove so they're out of reach.
- ✓ Turn off the pilot light on your gas fireplace. A baby or toddler who touches a lit gas fireplace will typically panic and press down harder on the hot glass rather than letting go, increasing the severity of the burn.
- ✓ Be aware that screens aren't strong enough to prevent a baby or child from falling out of a window, so make open windows inaccessible. Alternatively, install clips that limit how much windows can open.
- ✓ Keep dangerous chemicals and medications out of reach.
- ✓ Empty backyard wading pools when not in use.
- ✓ Close toilet lids. Toilets are also a drowning hazard.

- ✓ Cords from curtains, blinds, and exercise equipment can strangle a child; tie them up out of reach.
- ✓ Identify which house plants are poisonous.
- ✓ Make sure dressers, bookshelves, and other heavy furniture are fastened to the wall.
- ✓ Because choking can happen very quickly, don't let an unattended child have access to food.
- ✓ Install safety gates at the top and bottom of stairs.
- ✓ Make certain areas of your house physically off limits. It's easier to feel confident about your baby-proofing efforts if you focus on the parts of your home that you're okay with your child accessing on his own.

But do let your baby put that in his mouth.

Babies experience the world through their mouths. Some put things in their mouth more often than others, but all babies do it. It's an essential part of their growth and development. Instead of selecting toys based on colour, flashing lights, sounds, or claims about educational value, do your baby a solid and give him just one or two playthings selected on the basis of their chewability. Mouth feel is what matters most to him now.

See baby play!

Your baby is getting more interested in large objects he can grasp and chew, but there's no need to bring toys along if you're heading out the door. Wherever you're going, chances are there'll be ready entertainment for your baby. A grocery store, for example, has literally aisle after aisle after aisle of objects your baby has never seen before—a dangling mobile will just obstruct his view of these wonders. The local park has trees and leaves and squirrels. A dinner party is likely to have a houseful of people happy to cuddle and admire your pudgy little wudgykins.

The reason new parents tend to pack toys for every outing is because they assume, as baby becomes more alert to the outside world, that one of their jobs is to entertain him.

It isn't.

As a parent, you need to feed your baby and sleep your baby and change his diapers and tickle his tummy and tell him he's an absolute delight and introduce him to other people and noises and help him count his toes. But you don't need to entertain him. Nor is it your duty to *enrich* the mind of your progeny through forced one-on-one interaction. He doesn't need your pity play. You'll find it boring and—what's worse—your *baby* will find it boring, too.

If you're at a loss for what to "do" with your baby, stick him in a carrier and head out for a latte together. Then let him gnaw on the coffee lid.

CHAPTER 11:

Months 7 to 11

"He had just started to crawl, so this was a huge uptick in excitement for our time together. Prior to this, there was the watching my baby lie and the watching my baby eat. Now, with this new skill, there was the watching my baby crawl. It's not a huge thing, but weeks and weeks go by where very little happens, so even slight changes make a big difference in the day to day."

– From *Failure is an Option: An Attempted Memoir*, (2018) by H. Jon Benjamin

Keep nursing on demand throughout the day.

Nurse on demand and nurse "on offer."

While your baby may naturally be down to five or six nursing sessions per 24-hour period, it's still important to follow baby's lead on breastfeeding during the day.

Nursing should also be "on offer." Sometimes when babies become more mobile they get so busy that they accidentally skip a feeding. Be on the lookout for this. If your baby normally nurses five or six times per day and he suddenly dips down to three or four, consider taking him to a darkened room that has few distractions to offer him his milkie.

Babies continue to have a biological need for breastmilk at this age. In fact, if you were to wean your baby off breastmilk before 12 months, it wouldn't be a true weaning, because you'd have to replace nursing with bottles of a breastmilk substitute, such as formula. Babies are too young to subsist on solids alone at this age.

Your baby may stage a nursing strike.

Because babies under 12 months old are normally too young to wean, if yours suddenly and completely refuses the breast, you're likely dealing with what's called a "nursing strike." Nursing strikes typically last two to four days, but may last as long as ten days. With some internet searches and creativity, there's a very good chance you can figure out how to get past the nursing strike and back to breastfeeding.

Keep offering your baby solid foods.

> "For her first few months of eating solid foods, my youngest got a single sliver of a fresh red pepper for breakfast every morning while I was rushing to get her older siblings off to school. A vegetable for breakfast! I was too busy to think of anything else to toss at her tray and she was too young to object. So, it worked out for everybody."
>
> -Mom of Four

Once your baby is past the experimental first stages with solid foods, you can offer him two to three meals per day. Then, by the time he's 11 months old, you can ramp up to three or four meals per day (consisting of two to three fuller meals and one to two snacks between these bigger meals).

As he becomes more proficient at eating solid foods, try to find a component of each dish that you can offer to your baby as finger food and a component that you can mash up for spoon-feeding. This doesn't mean making the super-human effort to include a self-feeding and spoon-feeding item at *every* meal. It just means that you should look for naturally occurring *opportunities* at each meal to offer an item from each category.

Continue to combine spoon-feeding with offering finger foods as the mood strikes you, but be aware that at some point between seven and 11 months, your baby is likely to insist on taking over the spoon. When this happens, just roll with it.

For the first little while, your baby will be awkward and ineffective at feeding himself, but this is an important skill for him to learn. If he's enthusiastic about self-feeding, there's no need to temper that drive. And if you're worried he's not really getting anything in with his clumsy motor skills, then remember, "Under one, it's just for fun!" He's still getting lots of momma milk—more than you think—so this is the perfect stage to practise self-feeding.

And serve those meals exclusively at the table.

Whenever possible, serve your baby his two to four daily meals when he is seated at a table. Parents can quickly end up multiplying their child's daily meals by offering snacks on the go throughout the day. While it's ultimately up to you how often you choose to feed your baby, here are **four reasons** why you should consider skipping the snack-all-day, anytime-anywhere approach.

Reason #1: Eat-anywhere snacks tend to be unhealthy.

Snacks-on-the-go inevitably end up being carb-laden, sweetened, salted treats that sacrifice nutrition to minimize the stickiness and mess that tends to come with, say, a baby eating a ripe banana or soft peach. It's easier to accept stickiness and messiness at the table. Serving a soft peach on your shag carpet? *No bueno.*

Reason #2: Eat-anywhere unhealthy snacks end up replacing healthy food.

Non-messy snacks-on-the-go—such as cookies (read: Baby Num Nums), granola bars (not that far removed from chocolate bars), or dry cereal (lots of added sugar)—can create a reinforcing cycle. Baby quickly realizes that sugary, salty carbs are tastier than a well-balanced diet. So then baby gets fussier at table-time meals. So then parents panic that baby isn't getting enough to eat. So then parents offer more snacks between meals. Pretty soon you have a child who completely turns up his nose at carrots and broccoli but shovels in Baby Num Nums and Goldfish crackers with wild abandon.

Around the age of three, despite your best efforts, your child will become an incredibly picky eater—so take advantage of this brief window when he might be amenable to chewing on a steamed broccoli floret.

Reason #3: Feeding snacks then becomes your new job.

Once they gain the capacity to speak, all kids have an irritating tendency to pipe up with "I'm huuungry!" at frequent intervals. If you agree to feed your child *away* from the table, dealing with "I'm huuungry!" will go from a part-time aggravation to a full-time preoccupation. Soon your entire day will be spent doling out food to your child—15 calories at a time—to accommodate his growing desire for all-day cluster-feeding of snacks.

Here's the thing: snacks aren't breastmilk. You're under no obligation to dole out Baby Num Nums "on demand" as you do with breastmilk.

Reason #4: You'll start using food to placate your children.

Keeping a toddler quiet in public through a steady stream of Baby Num Nums is a gateway drug to handing over your smartphone to bribe that same child into remaining silent. Keeping meals at the table helps set the expectation that food is something we turn to when we're hungry, not bored.

Plus, with baby seated at a table, it'll be easier to introduce a cup with water.

Around the age of seven months or so, once solid foods are going well, you can start giving your baby the occasional sip of water.

There's no need to introduce a sippy cup.

Invented by Richard Belanger—a clever mechanical engineer and harried dad—in 1988 and sold by Playtex in the early 1990s, the sippy cup had a fabulous run with millennials back when they were babies. Alas, medical professionals no longer recommend sippy cups because babies who learn how to drink beverages from a sippy cup need to use a modified placement of their tongue, which can lead to speech problems down the road.

And while a sippy cup seems easier in the short term (because it eliminates the risk of spills), it's like giving a preschooler a bike with training wheels—it seems like an inevitability because so many people do it, but it ultimately prolongs the length of time it takes the child to master the skill and greatly increases the effort a parent needs to expend for the transition to happen.

A baby who's never used a sippy cup or bottle can easily figure out how to get really good at drinking from an open cup on his own well before the age of two. If he gets a sippy cup, on the other hand, it will take him longer to figure out how to use an open cup properly, because the mechanisms are so different. With a sippy cup a child has to tip his head all the way back and pour in the liquid. Ironically, there's no sipping involved. With an open cup, on the other hand, a child needs to just gently tip the cup and sip (yes, actually *sip!*) to move the beverage to his mouth. Mastering both techniques is complicated for a child—it's easier for toddlers to figure out how to drink out of just a regular, big-person-style, open cup and skip the sippy-cup stage altogether.

(Whether you want keep using the adult version—the kind that stops you from spilling your margarita at the beach—is another issue entirely.)[35]

For the first few months, your baby will need you to hold the cup and gently tip the rim towards his mouth.

Don't worry if he doesn't actually manage to sip anything the first few times he's offered water. At this point, he's just getting introduced to the idea of using a cup. He's already meeting his daily fluid needs with your breastmilk, so he's not thirsty. It may not seem like there's much breastmilk to be had at this age, but trust me: your baby is getting more than you think.

It's a messy process. Once your baby finally takes in the water, he'll struggle with where to place his tongue, and he'll sputter and cough. Liquid will spray everywhere. That's why, at this stage, you'll make your life easier if you offer water with just one meal per day. Not that there's harm in offering it with every meal, it's just that it's a chore. A single daily serving is good enough at this age because that solid-foods mantra—"under one, just for fun"—applies doubly to beverages. A baby under 12 months will end up taking in so little water that drinking from a cup is truly more for practice than hydration.

After around eight to nine months of age, once they enjoy taking in four or five sips, many (but not all) babies show interest in holding the cup on their own.

If yours is doing this, you need to let go of the cup, Momma. Let it go! Your hands can hover nearby to "spot" the whole process for the first few weeks, but let your baby work on this fine motor skill once he's keen to try.

---

[35] Editor's note: I once took apart one of our sippy cups and realized there was all this mould trapped inside, which is one of their design flaws. They're a perfect petri dish. Gross. See: themoldmedic.com/mold-in-sippy-cups-and-bottles-is-a-parenting-nightmare/

And if your baby shows no interest in holding the cup on his own, don't worry about it. He'll get there in his own good time.

And at this stage, water—not cow's milk—should be baby's beverage of choice.

Cow's milk would be too messy to offer in an open cup. But that's okay, because cow's milk isn't recommended in significant amounts until a baby is 12 months of age.

There's nothing special about cow's milk, anyway. Your goal, eventually, will be to replace breastmilk with your baby's *entire* well-balanced diet, and not just cow's milk. Cow's milk doesn't replace breastmilk. Carrots, water, beef, lettuce, Cheerios, bagels, cheesecake, tuna fish, snap peas, and cow's milk—collectively—replace breastmilk.

Respect your baby's need to sleep.

Your baby should continue to be a relatively predictable napper: going down around 9 am for at least one hour; going down around 1 pm for at least one hour; and going to sleep for the night around 6:30 pm.

On most days, your baby will go to sleep with either no tears or just a few minutes of light protest crying.

If your baby was taking a third nap—a late-afternoon or early-evening catnap—he'll likely phase it out at some point between months 7 and 11. There's nothing mom needs to do to phase out the third nap. Baby just stops falling asleep on his own. Dropping a nap tends to make a baby cranky, so be prepared with a backup plan: perhaps a trip to the park or some water play or a filling 4 pm snack.

When the third nap disappears, the remaining two naps tend to get a little longer and the wakeful time before the morning nap gets a little longer, too. This is why it's important to watch your baby for signs of sleepiness, and to avoid timing naptimes and bedtimes strictly by the clock. A 9 am naptime doesn't mean that the nap occurs at this exact hour—it just means you start watching your baby for slight fussing or a slowing in his movements around that time.

It's finally here: Your earliest opportunity for full, *parent*-led night-weaning.

Your baby was ready for partial night-weaning sometime between six and twelve weeks. However, at that age, some babies have a physiological need to nurse every four to six hours, so even if you partially night-weaned your baby a few months ago, he might still be waking once or twice a night to breastfeed (while babies who have not been partially night-weaned may be waking up three or four or more times a night to breastfeed).

The good news is that the physiological need that some babies have to feed at least every four to six hours at night doesn't continue after about nine months of age.

In other words, if your baby is at least nine months old and is regularly waking up at any point between his evening bedtime and his morning wake-up, you can now, if you like, night-wean him for this full, approximately 10-hour period.

Mercifully, sleep-training is usually the hardest the first time around. The second or third time around, leaving your baby to cry it out for just half an hour on a single night may be enough to lengthen his night sleep. (Remember to use a clock during the sleep-training process; otherwise, 30 minutes of crying might could feel like three hours.)

That being said, sleep-training can become agonizingly difficult if parents wait *too* long to do it. Once a toddler is old enough to crawl out of his big-boy bed and use his words to demand some nighttime parenting, you might be hooped. It takes more time, tears, and effort to night-wean the older your baby gets.

For help with night-weaning, see Chapter 7. The process for partial night-weaning and full night-weaning are exactly the same. The only difference is that with partial night-weaning you let baby make the call about whether any individual sleep period lasts longer than about four hours, whereas with full night-weaning you can coach baby into sleeping right through from his 6:30 pm(ish) bedtime until the morning.

If you're worried that parent-led night-weaning will harm your baby, rest assured that he's at a stage when momma's *need* for sleep can be placed ahead of baby's *wish* for milkie. After a baby is nine months old, a consistent pattern of night-waking occurs because baby hasn't had enough practice riding the sleep wave back into deeper slumber after hitting the "light non-REM" stage of sleep. It isn't due to hunger. Nor is it due loneliness, a fear of the dark, a fear of abandonment, or a sense of overwhelming dread. People aged two and up can have trouble sleeping due to anxiety, fear, and existential malaise—but not itty-bitty babies.

And, of course, night-weaning is always a family choice. If you prefer to continue night-nursing at this age, you can, for sure. When it comes to the decision about whether to night-wean, you're fine if you do and you're fine if you don't.

Screen time isn't recommended before age two.

Children can rarely walk at this age, but by 11 months most have figured out how to sit up on their own and then scooch on their bums or crawl on their hands and knees or step along with their feet while holding onto furniture.

At some point during this stage, your baby will also develop the gross motor skills to swipe through your iPhone. Impressive? Nah, not really. Obviously your baby *can*, but that doesn't mean he *should*. Screen time is not recommended for children under the age of two.

The rising ubiquity of babies using handheld devices can be partially traced, again, to misguided advice for parents to play with their babies. When a parent is told to play with her baby, then she assumes it's her job to keep her baby entertained. This means that the minute baby expresses displeasure, mom assumes she's not doing a good enough job with the entertainment. So then out pops the smartphone and baby's fussies melt away under the hypnotic spell of the screen.

But here's the thing: it's *not* your job to entertain your baby.

Your baby can entertain himself.

If baby is fussing and you can't get to him right now, either because you're busy trying to shower or racing to get the lasagna in the oven by a certain time, don't give him your cellphone. Just let him be. Let him fuss and figure out what to do about his own malaise or discomfort.

Human beings aren't meant to be placated every time we start airing our grievances. Your baby has the right to occasionally proclaim that he's feeling like a sour kangaroo.

Sometimes parents defend giving smartphones to babies and toddlers by exhorting others to cut them some slack. "It's the easiest way to get him to stop fussing," they may say.

I'm all for cutting parents some slack, but we need to redefine what that means. Rather than framing "no screen time before age two" as some sort of *Gold Standard* that only a mythical, perfect family could achieve, try to think of it this way: "I'm okay with both happy and unhappy emotions. My baby's fussing is age-appropriate, so, I'm going to cut *him* some slack."

Fortunately, 7- to 12-month-olds don't cry too much.

You shouldn't expect lots of crying at this stage; in large part because your baby's improved communication skills are making it easier for you to respond promptly to his needs. Around the age of seven months, babies become much better at controlling the pitch, tempo, and volume of their cries. They master what sleep researcher Dr. James McKenna calls "speech breathing," which means they can use different cries to communicate different needs. So instead of outright wailing, your baby is more likely to exhibit periods of mild fussiness. This is the age at which mommas get the boost of confidence that comes with being able to say, "Oh, he needs his naptime," or "It sounds like he's done with his food."

If you feel you're getting better at understanding what your baby is trying to tell you these days, it means you're actually pretty good at this, Momma. Sweet!

CHAPTER 12:

Months 12 to 15

"Motherhood is in many ways an exercise in varying degrees of freedom being granted or taken away. Occasionally you get offered what looks like a jailbreak — some magical new milestone in your child's life, like walking, or eating solids, or starting daycare that you imagine is going to free up x amount of time and let you regain some of your old autonomy. So you jump to take it — who wouldn't? — only to find yourself not celebrating, not rejoicing, but sitting around missing what you just gave up."

—Tracy Moore (2012)[36]

New development: *Momma* gets to decide when to nurse!

You did it! You're past the stage when you need to nurse your baby on demand!

After 12 months of nursing "on demand," it can be a bit of an adjustment: Baby no longer calls the shots. From now on, day or night, it's

---

[36] From "No, You're Not Pregnant and Simultaneously PMSing, You Just Weaned a Toddler" (August 23, 2012), available at: jezebel.com/no-you-re-not-pregnant-and-simultaneously-pmsing-you-5937022

you who decides whether to nurse. While your baby still benefits from the breastmilk he gets at this age, you now have the final say on when breastfeeding happens at any time, day or night.

Two things can trip up moms at this stage of breastfeeding:

1. The desire to keep weaning "natural" by continuing to nurse on baby's demand.
2. The desire to wean baby cold turkey as soon as he hits the magical age of 12 months.

Let's get into these two concepts in more detail.

Potential trip-up #1: The desire to keep weaning "natural"

Every family's experience is different. I suppose it is possible, in the realm of hypothetical possibilities, for mom to continue following her child's lead on breastfeeding until both are ready to quit at exactly the same time.

The reality is much messier.

If you strive for a so-called "natural" weaning and let your toddler continue to nurse on demand, you run the risk of setting unrealistic expectations that end in frustration and tears—for both of you.

Potential trip-up #2: The desire to wean baby entirely as soon as he hits 12 months.

When baby is a year old, you may start feeling pressure to wean him entirely. Maybe you, your husband, your mother-in-law, or your best friend have never met a baby who was nursed into toddlerhood. Maybe you just assumed—without thinking too much about it—that babies wean before they're out of diapers.

But an abrupt weaning can be hard on baby and momma. Babies between the ages of one and two who are getting average amounts of mother's milk receive 35 to 40 percent of their food intake from it. That's a lot of calories to cut out cold turkey!

Plus, this stage—12 to 15 months—can be a particularly difficult time to abruptly cut off nursing because there's so much going on for baby. He's working on walking and talking[37] and maybe dropping his morning nap and climbing playground equipment and making his first attempts at imaginative play. If you add an abrupt weaning to all of this, it can just feel like too much.

Weaning is easier without a specific date in mind.

Rather than go hog-wild on either scenario—continued nursing-on-demand or quitting cold turkey—you can make the process easier on both you and baby by landing somewhere in the middle and gently encouraging baby to nurse less often after the age of 12 months.

For starters, consider cutting out a nursing session the next time baby drops a nap.

Now that he's over the age of one, your baby will likely drop another of his daytime naps. He probably already dropped his third nap (if he was having one) a few weeks ago. At some point between 12 and 18 months, most babies drop the morning nap, too. Once yours makes this transition, you'll have a golden opportunity to cut out the nursing session, or sessions, associated with that nap. (Some babies nurse to fall asleep, some nurse as soon as they wake up, and some do both.)

Be aware, though, that many babies want to nurse *more* once they've dropped the morning nap, because they feel unsettled by the large reduction in sleep. Suddenly your baby will be awake for longer, which means more hours to fill, which can lead to a new feeling: boredom. What's a bored, cantankerous, no-nap baby to do? He knows the answer: *Breastfeed!*

Remember, Momma, now that your baby is over 12 months old, *you* get to set the parameters for the amount of breastfeeding you will and will not allow. There are plenty of fun ways to distract a toddler

---

[37] Most children learn their first word around the age of 12 months. By 16 to 18 months, most have expanded their vocabulary to about 50 words!

and take his mind off his milko. You're ready to reach for the other tools in your tool belt.

Also, feel free to cut a nursing session *short* if you're not into it.

You know how many (not all) moms get a rush of feel-good hormones when they're nursing a newborn baby? Well the opposite can happen at this stage. The feelings that some moms experience while breastfeeding a child over 12 months old run from irritation, resentment, "nails on a chalkboard," to physical annoyance at having one's nipple pulled in baby's mouth. These feelings are unpleasant to experience, but also perfectly normal. If breastfeeding is giving you the heebie jeebies, you're not obligated to make a martyr out of yourself. Simply put your finger in baby's mouth to unlatch him.

This should ideally be a tear-free process. If you unlatch baby and he starts to cry, you can try to soothe away his tears by distracting him: sticking him in a baby carrier, cuddling him on your lap and reading a book, or taking him to the playground.

Don't worry about replacing breastfeeding sessions if you're back at work.

Whoever is caring for your baby while you're at work is probably a pro with a big bag of tricks for getting babies to fall asleep. And if it's your partner and you assume he has no bag of tricks and doesn't exactly strike you as a pro—don't worry about that either. He's a parent. He's got this. Let your baby's caregiver figure out how to soothe him to sleep.

There's no need to pump breastmilk for your baby who is over 12 months old.

Nursing at the breast is as much for baby's comfort as it is for nutrition, so you might as well let your caregiver comfort him in whatever way works.

At this stage, your body and your baby can adjust to the missed breastfeeding sessions.

To give you an idea of what happens when you abruptly stop nursing your 12- to 15-month-old baby for 8-10 hours per day when you return to work, I've created an outline of a typical week below. I've based it on Monday to Friday, the most common work schedule, but of course, adjust as necessary to reflect your own.

Here's what your week may look like:

Monday.

- Nurse your toddler before you go to work in the morning.

- Let your caregiver feed him solids and offer him a cup of water throughout the day. Have faith that your caregivers will find their own methods to soothe your toddler down for his nap.

- You'll likely find that, as the day goes on, your breasts get fuller and fuller, so it's a good idea to wear breast pads to work for the first few weeks back. If someone mentions "baby" near the end of the day, you may need to subtly squeeze your forearms against your breasts to prevent an embarrassing letdown!

- When you and your baby are reunited at the end of the day he'll likely want to nurse and nurse and nurse. Some moms (just some) find this a welcome way to reconnect. Most find it downright irritating; your brain is still sort of in work mode, you haven't yet had time to make dinner, and you just want to crawl into bed and have some alone time for a few minutes. It can help to know that babies tend to have this intense need to be held by mom after work regardless of whether they are breastfeeding, so weaning won't necessarily solve the problem if you find this particular after-work ritual annoying. You're better off recognizing that it's normal baby behaviour and accepting that you'll likely need to devote 45 minutes after work every day to giving your toddler the momma-time he craves.

- In the evening, do your normal routine of nursing your toddler to sleep.

Tuesday to Friday.

- Repeat all the above.
- As the week progresses, you'll find that your breasts feel less and less full. If on Friday someone mentions "baby" at work, you might have no letdown at all.

The weekend.

- You can go back to your old, pre-return-to-work breastfeeding routine. Feel free to nurse him down for every nap, and to nurse him throughout the day whenever you feel like it.
- On Monday your breastmilk supply will be right back up again, and you'll again run the risk of a letdown by late afternoon.

After a few weeks back at work, your breasts will catch on to what's happening, and you'll stop running the risk of a letdown emergency in the late afternoon on Mondays. That said, it might take a few months before your baby lets go of his intense need for momma-time after work.

While spending this much time away from baby would have destroyed your milk supply back when he was 12 *weeks* old, after 12 *months*, milk supply becomes incredibly resilient, going up and down with baby's needs. This is why it's not necessary to do any special weaning when you return to work after around 12 months of parental leave.[38] Your body just naturally adjusts throughout the week. Pretty amazing, eh?

---

38 If you live in a jurisdiction where parental leave ends much sooner, have a look at the resources listed in the "Breastfeeding" section at the end of this book. Many American writers and bloggers have useful information about breastfeeding and returning to work when baby is a few weeks old.

Your baby is also quite flexible about breastfeeding at this stage. He clearly knows the difference between when momma is around and when momma is away. When momma is with him, he wants his usual milkie. When another caregiver is in charge, he's fine with solid foods and cups of water for meals and soothing back rubs and lullabies for bedtime.

Don't worry about replacing breastfeeding if you go out for the evening, either.

For example, let's say you're planning to go out for dinner at 5:30 pm, but baby's bedtime is 6:30 pm. No problem! All you need to do is nurse baby before leaving—say around 5 pm, right after he's had his solid-foods dinner. Of course, he won't fall asleep this early, but at least you'll feel reassured that he got his milko. Then leave him with an experienced babysitter and go on your dinner date.

I say "experienced babysitter" because if you're not there at bedtime and baby is used to nursing to sleep, there *will* be crying involved. It's fine to hire an 11-year-old babysitter for most of your evening outings, but caring for baby when there's a difficult bedtime involved is a situation that requires an experienced set of hands, like a grandparent or an adult nanny. Just let your caregivers know the deal—baby normally nurses down to sleep, but not tonight—and they'll figure out their own way of soothing him to bed.

If you give your babysitters a heads up that baby's likely to be upset, then they'll be prepared. Maybe they'll jiggle baby and sing to him softly. Maybe they'll cuddle him and read him stories. Maybe they'll let him fall asleep crying in their arms. It takes a bit of work, but it won't be as bad as when you were sleep-training. We're taking about 10 to 30 minutes of crying—not hours—and with someone soothing him the whole time.

Even if you feel guilty, there's absolutely no need to change your plans. It's healthy for mom to go out. It's healthy for babies to go without their milkie occasionally at this age. Everyone wins!

And the good news for baby is that you can nurse him down to sleep tomorrow. Mother Nature designed our bodies to be flexible at this stage of breastfeeding.

Figure out what to tell your mother-in-law/sister/best friend/neighbour when they say, "What?! You're still nursing?!"

To begin with, plenty of mothers nurse children past the age of one. It's just that others aren't always aware of it because the nursing typically happens only at home—either to fall asleep or shortly after waking up—which means babies are tucked away in a bedroom while breastfeeding, where no outsiders get to see them.

But even though it's typical to do less public nursing at this age, you may still find yourself outed about breastfeeding your toddler. If someone registers surprise (or raises an objection), the first thing you need to do, Momma, is take a deep breath. The reason this person made a comment is because he or she genuinely cares about your child. While the unsolicited[39] comment might be putting you in the red zone, take a pause. A big pause.

Breathe in.

Breathe out.

Getting testy with people is not a good way to effect change, so lead with gratitude for the person's caring.

After you've taken a deep, deep breath, here are a few ideas for how to respond:

- "The World Health Organization and my doctor recommend nursing for two years and beyond."

- "I didn't realize that toddlers still nurse at this age either. I thought he'd be out of diapers by now, too. It turns out most toddlers continue to wear diapers (and nurse) well into their second year of life. Diapers and breastfeeding—both

---

39 Unsolicited: the worst form of comment, observation, suggestion or advice.

age-appropriate. I guess they're still closer to being babies than big kids at this age!"

- "It's true—a baby no longer needs breastmilk at this age. Now that he's 12 months old, if I were to wean him, I wouldn't need to replace the breastmilk with formula. He could just go without it. But while it's no longer necessary, it's still nutritious and beneficial for him. Think of carrots. The fibre, the vitamin C, and the beta carotene that our bodies convert into vitamin A—we get all of this from carrots. Baby could easily get the same nutritional benefits from other foods. But why cut out carrots when they're good for him? Same with breastmilk. He's lucky to have this easy source of probiotics and nutrients, including fatty acids, vitamin A, calcium, and riboflavin. Why deny him the good stuff?"

- "I've seen kids this age with bottles. This is basically the same thing."

- "I've seen kids this age walk around with soothers in their mouth. This is basically the same thing."

- "I remember when you were this age you used to walk around with your thumb in your mouth and your blankie. This is basically the same thing."[40]

- "It sounds like you're bringing this up because you're concerned about whether we're doing the right thing for our baby. I'm glad he's got you in his corner. I'll email you some information so you can read about the benefits of breastfeeding at this age. But really, bottom line, I'm glad you spoke up, because it means you're one of the people who cares about our little pumpkin."

---

40 Might be getting too personal and bitter with this one. Right: Breathe in. Breathe out.

Which brings me to another possibility: Consider that maybe, just maybe, the concerned family member or friend has a valid point. Now, obviously, nursing past the age of 12 months is healthy for a child and recommended by health professionals and all that, but whenever a friend or family member makes a comment about any aspect of your parenting, consider that they may just have a legitimate kernel of wisdom to pass on.

The people closest to us and our children know us best. Not as well as we know ourselves, to be sure, but they sometimes notice when we're acting in a self-defeating manner.

So, go ahead and bristle when a concerned (read: interfering) busybody tells you that you're breastfeeding too often or disciplining too seldom. But then mull over their words with an open mind. Maybe there's some aspect of what you're doing that could benefit from a little adjustment?

Finally, if you're feeling anxious or upset about another person's take on breastfeeding, turn to your tribe of like-minded mommas. It's unrealistic to take on the gargantuan task of convincing all family members, friends, neighbours, and strangers that this is what the normal course of breastfeeding looks like. Protecting your child's right to breastfeed matters—but your relationships with the people around you matter, too. Talking with friends about a difficult encounter can help relieve tension and renew your confidence.

Keep offering your baby solid foods.

Expect a total of five to six sittings at the table per day.

Your baby could be up to three or four larger meals per day at this stage, with one or two smaller snacks in-between, making for a total of five to six sittings at the table per day. If he still has both a morning and afternoon nap, you can expect the total number of meals (including snacks) to be closer to between four and five per day. After your child has dropped the morning nap, which will give him more free time in his day, the number of meals he eats should inch up to between five and six per day.

Meal timing

Expect the timing of your toddler's meals to roughly correspond with: (1) breakfast; (2) a possible morning snack; (3) lunch; (4) a 4:30 pm substantial snack or early dinner; and, (5) possibly an evening snack or second dinner.

Many babies eat two dinners at this stage because they're hungry well before the rest of the family is ready to eat, and then they're ready for a little bit more when the family sits down for the evening meal. (Pro tip: Some parents save leftovers from the previous evening to serve to baby around 4:30 pm.)

Most babies have taken over spoon-feeding by now.

In the normal course of introducing solid foods, by the time a baby is 12 months old, he no longer needs to be spoon-fed by an adult. He can fully spoon-feed and finger-feed himself.

Watch sugar intake by treating special treats as a special treat.

In December 2020, the US government issued dietary guidelines that recommend **no added sugar** whatsoever for children under two.[41] Most kids are significantly exceeding these amounts.

To manage your children's sugar intake, learn how to read ingredient labels for added sugar. A lot of supposedly healthy snacks are no better than cookies or candy bars. Culprits include flavoured yogurt tubes, baby crackers, fruit juice, many breakfast cereals, and most granola bars. Savoury food items—such as pasta sauces, frozen meals, and deli meats—can also have added sugar where none is necessary.

---

[41] Available at: cdc.gov/nutrition/infantandtoddlernutrition/. For kids over two, the World Health Organization, the American Heart Association, and Canada's Heart and Stroke Foundation have all called for a daily maximum of six teaspoons of added sugar for kids (and a maximum of ten teaspoons for adults).

If you take the time to read and compare ingredient labels when you're grocery shopping, you can pick out the healthiest choices for your family. But it's no easy task. Even vigilant shoppers have trouble interpreting the presence or level of added sugar because there are currently 152 different ways to list sugar without calling it sugar on food labels. Some key words to look for: glucose, fructose, maltose, dextrose, fruit concentrates, fruit juice concentrates, fruit purees, fruit evaporates, honey, maltodextrin, dehydrated cane juice, cane syrup, barley malt syrup, brown rice syrup, and potato syrup solids.

If you also want to minimize *artificial* sweeteners in your baby's diet, key words to look for include: aspartame, sucralose, acesulfame potassium, or the red-herring phrase "no sugar added" (followed by an artificial sweetener listed in the ingredients list).

> **Pro tip:**
>
> Many families avoid dessert until baby's first birthday.
>
> Being the centre of attention with a large slice of birthday cake, with photos snapped to mark the occasion, balloons, streamers, fanfare, and singing—what a delightful introduction to the deliciousness of desserts!

Another way to manage your toddler's sugar intake is to keep the emphasis on *fun*. Sugary indulgences should be consumed as a treat during life's big events. Sweet things for Halloween, birthday parties, and Sunday dinners are delightful. The risk of overconsumption increases when sugary treats are tossed in the mix every day.

Brush your baby's teeth.

As soon as baby's first tooth appears you can begin to brush it—especially before bedtime—with a soft-bristled baby toothbrush. When baby is 12 months you can add a small amount of child-friendly toothpaste—the size of a cooked grain of rice.

New development: Baby drops the morning nap.

You were doing so well with the napping. You knew the routine inside out. You'd nailed it!

Then just as you were really getting into the groove, your baby goes and stages a revolt.

This is a heads up for you, Momma: At some point soon[42] your baby's going to drop one of his two major daytime naps.

Just to be clear—eliminating daytime naps is something your baby will do **on his own**. He doesn't need any parental help with this. In fact, you don't *want* to do anything to speed along this process. You want—*you desperately want*—him to nap for as long as possible.

Once he decides, on his own, that it's time to drop one of his two major daytime naps, there are two ways he'll go about it. Let's go over each scenario.

Scenario #1: You're a lucky, lucky momma. Your by-the-book baby drops the morning nap.

The gold standard is that your baby—your clever, clever little baby—drops the morning nap all by himself.

Sometimes people ask, "Do you have a good baby?" A baby who drops the morning nap on his own probably deserves an affirmative response to this question: "Yes, I *do* have a good baby."

This is how it'll go down. Sometime around this age, you'll nurse baby down as usual for his morning nap and put him in his crib. But then one of two things will happen.

A. **Baby won't fall asleep.** He'll stay awake and keep babbling. And if you leave him in the crib, he'll start to cry! Since we're not at a sleep-training stage, there's nothing to be gained by leaving baby in his crib to cry for too long. If he's crying for more than ten

---

[42] While I've put this drop-the-nap information in the "12 to 15 Months Old" section, some babies drop their morning nap as early as 10 to 12 months of age, while others keep going strong with two naps per day for 18 months or longer. It's perfectly normal if this section doesn't apply to your baby yet.

minutes, just go and get him. He's clearly not going to fall asleep this morning.

B. **Baby falls asleep but wakes up a short while later.** If your baby over the age of 12 months cuts short his morning nap, there's nothing to be gained by leaving him in his crib to cry. Just go and get him. Naptime is done for the morning.

This no-nap or short-nap could be a one-off occurrence, so try again tomorrow to put him down for his morning nap.

But if he resists it for a week straight, it's safe to say your baby has dropped the morning nap.

If that's the case, you may need to start serving lunch earlier—say 10:30 or 11 am, because he may be ready for his afternoon nap before noon. You may also want to serve a morning snack around 9 am to distract him from mid-morning teariness and irritability. In transitioning from two naps to one, there's a difficult adjustment period where "two is too many and one is not enough."

Scenario #2: Not so lucky. Your baby drops the afternoon nap.

So your baby didn't get the memo about dropping the morning nap first.

Some babies drop the *afternoon* nap first, while the morning nap is still going strong. If your baby resists the afternoon nap for a week straight, it's safe to say he's now dropped it.

Bad, bad baby.

If your baby eliminates his afternoon nap, you're in for a world of hurt, because he's never going to make it all the way from his late-morning wake-up to his 6:30 pm bedtime without a meltdown. You, my dear, *are* going to have a persnickety baby on your hands in the afternoon.

Worst: there's *nothing* you can do about it.

Oh, sure, the internet may tell you to move his morning nap up by 15 minutes over the next few weeks, to which I say: Bollocks! You can keep trying to inch up his nap, but it will be a struggle. Every. Single. Day. You can attempt every suggestion the internet throws at you to keep him awake—introducing a morning snack, singing to him, doing patty-cake rhymes, reading stories, going for playdates—but you'll likely just end up with a fussy baby who conks out like clockwork for a 9 am snooze.

You'll also have to deal with a cranky baby in the afternoon who just won't sleep. Cranky baby: no fun. And no fair—since the moms whose babies dropped their morning nap don't have to deal with this aggravation.

If your baby is cranky in the afternoon, one option is to stick him in a carrier. He may eventually be lulled into taking a 20-minute catnap while you walk, which will at least buy you a little peace. Another method that works in rare cases is to wake up your baby from his morning nap after just one hour. He may then be willing to go down for another hour in the afternoon. (But I doubt it.)

Bottom line: No matter what you do you'll still have to deal with a fussy, cranky baby.

sigh

If yours is one of those rare babies who drops the afternoon nap and keeps the morning nap, there is one ray of hope. Most babies follow the same developmental stages most of the time, so chances are that eventually, *on his own*, your baby will move his single nap to the afternoon. May the odds be ever in your favour.

At this stage, if baby is fussy, respond to him—*sometimes.*

At this age, many babies begin to *cry* less and *shriek* more. They're irritated about losing the morning nap. They're mobile enough to fling themselves on the floor, with four limbs pounding, but not yet functionally verbal. They never get their way on anything, or so it seems to them. What parents end up with are lots of meltdowns. Non-stop meltdowns. Conventional wisdom has it that the "terrible twos" are the toughest stage of parenting, but many moms and dads find the period between 12 and 15 months the most frustrating. Trying to interpret the piercing, wordless demands of a *verklempt* one-year-old can shatter anyone's sanity.

A nugget of wisdom from parents who have been there before you: *Respond to your toddler, but not too much.*

After all, you now have a greater, more comprehensive set of tools to reach for when your toddler is crying. It's a toolbox that includes—meaning it's not your only option—picking up your grumpy wumpy for a cuddle or a nursing. When your child is firing on all cylinders, just keep digging around until you find the right tool. It's got to be in there somewhere…

Twelve parent-tested tricks to tame toddler tantrums.

Tool #1: Food.

Adults don't eat as often as toddlers, so it's easy to forget that a rumbly in his tumbly could be making him grumbly.

Tool #2: Sleep.

Remember, crying is one of your toddler's only tools for communication, so he's using it to express a wide variety of needs. Don't automatically assume he's trying to tell you, "I need cuddles or milkie." He might just be trying to say, "I'm tired!"

Tool #3: Add water.

> "The cure for anything is salt water: sweat, tears or the sea."
>
> — Baroness Karen Christenze Blixen-Finecke, writing under pen name Isak Dineson in 1934 (1885–1962)

If it's cold out, run a warm bath in your house. If it's nice out, give your child a chance to splash around in a toddler pool or sprinkler. It's amazing how quickly water play can make a toddler forget about his troubles.

Tool #4: Take him outside.

There's a daily period between 3 and 8 pm when little kids seem to need A-level parenting. They've had a long day and they're at a point when any trifling disappointment can push them over the edge. Experienced moms know that 4 pm isn't the time to make dinner or try to get chores done. It's park time!

Shortly after learning to walk, your toddler will begin to master playground equipment, so this is a great age to make park visits a regular part of your routine.

And the fresh air, sunshine, trees, rocks, and other natural elements he'll connect with outside can quite literally make your harried little human being feel grounded. Scientists even have discovered a bacteria in soil, *mycobacterium vaccae*, that helps our bodies produce serotonin, which in turn helps our bodies enter a "rest and digest" state (the opposite of "fight or flight"). Getting down and dirty is a natural upper!

According to experts, children of all ages should have a minimum of two to three hours outdoor play time each day, so if you haven't yet met today's quota and your toddler is cranky, try heading outside.

Tool #5: Name it to tame it.

If your child has a tantrum in response to you saying "no" to a request, try this handy trick: use words to name the pain. Kids often shriek at this age because they urgently want to tell you something, but they don't have the vocabulary. Once your toddler knows you've heard him, he may turn off the escalating emergency alarm—the one that triggered his primitive limbic system into raising his heart rate, breathing rate, and blood pressure.

Let's say your toddler was playing with some marbles (choking hazard!), which you've taken away. He begins to sob. So you say, "Wow, you sound very upset. I can tell that you're *mad* because mommy took away the marbles. You want the marbles back. You really, really wish mommy would give you the marbles."

Amazingly, this trick can actually work. Really! A toddler will sometimes stop melting down once they hear that you've understood what they wanted—even if they don't get the item they're demanding! The toddler brain is *remarkable*.

Tool #6: Defer to a higher authority.

Another trick involves deferring to a higher power.

For example: "You really hate wearing a sun hat to the park. I hate wearing one, too. But the doctor says we're not allowed to play outside in the sunshine without a sun hat on."

Or: "I hate wearing a seatbelt, too. But the policeman says we have to do it."

You can also pretend to defer to an invented authority's arbitrarily set rules. "You want to visit another section of the zoo? I'd love that, too, but we can't. The zoo says we can only visit three sections today. We'll have to see the penguin exhibit next time."

If you insist the decision is out of your hands, then your sobbing toddler may conclude that there's no use lobbying *you* for a change in policy.

Tool #7: Fill your kid in on what's going to happen next.

If prevention is worth a pound of cure, then one of the best tools you have is talking to your toddler.

Often, in our rush to get from one thing to the next, we forget that our kids may not be up to speed on what's happening. Even at 12 months, kids are less likely to lose it if you give them a heads up along the lines of: "We're going to put your shoes on and then we're going to daycare!"

"I signed us up for Mommy and Me Swim Time. We'll go every week! I'm going to bring this swim bag and when we get there I will change you into a swimsuit."

"We have to leave the playground in 10 minutes."

Communicating clearly isn't only about letting your kids know that something new is about to happen. It's also about helping them understand what's happening in the moment. For example, even if you gave a 10-minute warning, don't just grab your child and leave. Instead, use your words: "I know you're having fun at the park, but *now* we are going to go home."

Tool #8: Press CTRL-ALT-DELETE and do a hard reboot. Then offer a choice between two things at the very end.

If your toddler has ramped up the drama, and you have a long list of tasks to do, take a deep breath, and work your sobbing, blubbering child through as many of the tasks as possible, and then, at (or near) the very end, let him choose between two options that are acceptable to you. When you're done the series of things you really needed to get done, then—and only then—invent something—anything—that returns to him his power to make decisions.

For example, let's say its bedtime. You take him to bed. He says, "No!" He starts kicking and screaming. When little children experience what might seem to you like an easily surmounted frustration, their feelings can become very, very *intense*!

Take a deep breath and stick with your plan. Calmly take your toddler up to bed (as he resists by going limp), calmly change his diaper (as he wriggles and fights), and calmly stick some pajamas on him (as he continues to sob). Do all this as quickly as you can, and all while he continues to loudly protest.

Then, when you're done with the core parts of the bedtime routine, as your toddler continues to rage against the parental machine, offer him two choices where you truly don't care what he picks. "Do you want water in this cup? Or in *this* cup?" "Do you want a book today? Yes? No?"

Your toddler may still be crying at this point, but the intensity may be starting to drop.

Show him that you're listening to his choices but be flexible if he changes his mind. Because he's already outraged by how unfair life is, there's a good chance he'll just shout "no!" regardless of what you suggest. You can respect his "no," at least initially: "What? No book today? Ok, bye, bye."

But also, give him an opportunity to reboot. Come back if he changes his mind and starts shouting, "Book! Book!"

Keep letting him choose between two non-consequential options until you find one that succeeds in distracting him. "Do you want mommy to pick the book? Or do *you* want to pick the book?" "Do you want *two* books? Or do you want *three* books?"

After book and cuddle times are done, you can say, "Do you want mommy to turn out the light or do *you* want to turn out the light?" By this point, the majority of toddlers will have completely calmed down.

The "pick-one-of-two-choices" technique works because it distracts your toddler and gives him that good feeling of control over what's happening to him. But it doesn't work if you offer it too early in a multi-step process, especially if there are "must-do" things that you know your child will object to. *First*, do what absolutely must be done, and *then* give him some limited control.

Sometimes toddlers can "reset" if they get control over a new decision—and they'll miraculously forget all about the previous issue where they didn't get their way. At times the limited brain power of toddlers can be maddening. Other times you can use it to outsmart them.

Tool #9: Take back the iPad. Turn off the TV.

Pediatricians, obesity researchers, and other experts recommend no TV, no iPad, no smartphone, no tablet– no screen time of any kind— before 24 months of age.

None.

Zero.

Nada.

Now this isn't because there is something inherently wrong with screen time. Digital devices have proven benefits. They're fun, they're entertaining, and they make life more convenient. For adults they're downright indispensable. But there's also a growing body of evidence that digital devices can have harmful effects on babies and toddlers. For children under two, no screen time is best.

Fortunately, avoiding screen time is simple, particularly if you avoid it 100 percent of the time. If you want your child under 24 months not to have screen time, what you do is this: you don't provide your child with screen time before the age of 24 months. It really is that simple.

As a parent, you have the power. If 75 percent of the parents around you are giving their toddlers screen time, then 25 percent are making it a non-starter. You can be part of the 25 percent.

All human beings get worn down by prodding. Once you've put screen time within the realm of possibility, your baby won't give up on asking for it. And because every parent gets tired of saying "No," you'll inevitably reach that moment of exhaustion when it's easier to comply than resist.

This is why delaying the onset of screen time is a whole lot easier than trying to "manage" it once the floodgates are opened. The hard truth is that no parent has the emotional fortitude to limit screen time, even if they say they do. Any parent who says "We only allow 20 minutes per day" or "Our kids get no more than two hours per week" is stretching the truth of what actually happens. Once you go down the path of allowing TV time or iPhone time or iPad time, you'll forever have to deal with an exhausting chorus of "I want that," "I want that," "I want that."

And you'll end up giving in far more often than you think.

Perhaps passing an iPhone to a toddler will one day become as deeply unnatural as lighting up a cigarette in a child's playroom. For the present moment, however, our Stone-Aged decision-making system is failing to ring any alarm bells. The only way around this is a system override: Let your controlled, rational, prefrontal cortex make the call and tame your toddler's tantrums by keeping him away from digital devices.

Tool #10: Consider a cuddle or story time.

Small children love to be picked up and held. It's one of their favourite things in the world. If your toddler or preschooler is getting fussy, you can pick him up and read to him or cuddle until he's ready to play again. Or you can stick him in a baby carrier and bring him along for whatever you're doing, whether it's walking the dog or making dinner. Holding your child close reassures him that he's surrounded by caring adults who adore him.

Tool #11: Get busy with your momma stuff.

I don't know why this magical momma trick works, but it does. If your toddler is fussy and demanding your attention but you've already done the pick-up-and-cuddle thing a few times and it's driving you to the brink of insanity, then find a very busy, very active momma task. Reading the paper or working on your laptop won't cut it. A toddler will see that as an opportunity to sniffle and tug on your sleeve and try to distract you some more. No, find something truly active: maybe chopping up things for dinner at the kitchen counter or assembling Ikea furniture.

Focus on your task. Step over your wailing child as you go about your busy work, give him occasional eye contact and a reassuring smile, help match words to his feelings ("Wow, you sound really upset. I bet you wish momma could play zoom-zoom cars with you. But I need to assemble this Ikea cabinet right now")—and continue doing what you need to do.

In a few minutes the caterwauling will turn to sniffles and then the sniffles will turn to him listlessly rolling a stray toy car around the kitchen floor, and then absentminded rolling will turn into contented, self-directed playtime. Really! It's like magic. Parental bustling and busywork somehow helps one- or two-year-olds regroup and reset their brains.

Tool #12. Do nothing.

Even though it's the last suggestion on this list, keep the do-nothing option top of mind as one of your tools. While you don't want to leave your baby to cry for no reason, as he moves through his toddler years there will be many circumstances when your job will still be to soothe away his tears, but also occasional circumstances when your job will be to *manage your own anxiety* about his crying.

All of us—even toddlers—need the opportunity to just vent sometimes. Imagine how frustrated you'd feel if someone tried to make you stop crying or prevented you from expressing your outrage every time you were upset. Sometimes we feel sad or mad—those are legitimate feelings—and sometimes crying legitimately helps.[43]

If you've already amply demonstrated to your child that he's surrounded by the people who love him most, then don't worry about occasionally giving him some space. Sometimes a child who's been bottling up all sort of big feelings just needs to let it all out.

And cry.

Here, once again, is an aspect of parenting that's more art than science. On the one hand, healthy attachment won't make your baby over-clingy. In fact, it will have the opposite effect. Your warmth and responsiveness will make baby feel secure and calm. And yet. There are parents who take responsiveness to such an extreme that their toddlers are constantly clingy and crying and pawing to be picked up or nursed.

This 12-to-15-months stage is where the invalidated tidbit may have been born: "Don't keep picking up your baby every time he cries; you'll spoil him." Dr. Spock and numerous other parenting theorists have correctly pointed out that applying this mantra to the infant stage is misguided and dangerous. What may have been lost, however, is that it's actually not bad advice for the baby who is old enough to walk and maybe talk. It's not true that you shouldn't pick up your baby. What may be true is this: Don't keep picking up your *toddler* every time he cries. Sometimes you can give it a minute.

---

43 It really does. A biochemical analysis of tears found an endorphin named leucine-enkephalin that's known to reduce pain and improve mood.

CHAPTER 13:

Months 16 to 24

"The park, in NYC, is basically a second home for child-rearing. A good part of early childhood is spent in parks. And a community forms among those who populate the parks. It's where moms and dads and their children form early bonds. It is also where early petty resentments develop. The park is a breeding ground for parents to judge other parents and develop private animosities toward them, the caregivers, and the children….The park is also a forum for public judgment on how children are raised, and many are not shy about sharing opinions. I wasn't immune to this…I judged parents for being overly precious about their babies. I judged parents who spoke harshly to other people's children. I pushed theories of parenting that I knew very little about."

—From *Failure is an Option: An Attempted Memoir*, (2018) by H. Jon Benjamin

Breastfeed if you want to; wean if you want to.

While both momma and baby still benefit from breastfeeding at this age, remember that you no longer need to nurse on demand.

If your toddler wants to nurse more often than you do, here are five ideas to gently reduce the amount of breastfeeding that happens:

- ✓ **Make rules.** Make up an arbitrary rule that works for you and then stick to it. The rule itself is totally up to you. Some examples: "only at night," "only in the daytime," "only at home," "only when we're cuddled on the one special chair," "never on the chesterfield," "only at bedtime." This way you can always remind your child (and yourself) of the rules and pretend you have no control over the matter. Lie blatantly: "Golly gumdrops, I would love to nurse you right now, but you know the rules: Only in the special chair! And our special chair isn't at the park. That's just the rule. It's out of my hands!"
- ✓ **Positive procrastination.** "Yes, of course, later."
- ✓ **Make the nursing shorter.** Put your finger in his mouth to break the suction then unlatch him.
- ✓ **Distraction.** "Who wants to colour!?" "Let's go sledding!"
- ✓ **Introduce a new soothing-to-sleep routine.** For example, read one story together in a special chair, then hold baby and sway gently while singing a lullaby, then place him in his crib and spend a few minutes slowly rubbing his belly or his back. You can also try stroking the top of his head by gliding your fingertips up his forehead and into his hair.

It's up to you whether to try these any of these tips to cut down on nursing. You know best what works for your family.

If you want to more actively encourage weaning, make it your goal to cut out just one nursing at a time.

Rather than aiming for a full weaning by a certain date, focus on mini goals (and mini wins!) that involve eliminating just one nursing at a time

Start with the easiest-to-cut-out nursing session first.

For many babies, the soothing-to-bed nursing at night matters most. So if you know that the "nurse me down to sleep" nursing is the one your child needs more than anything else in his day, then leave that one for last. Start by trying to eliminate the nursing you think he'll miss the least, then work your way up.

For the *majority* of babies, gradual weaning works at this age.[44]

Every time you successfully cut out a nursing session, work on cutting out the next one in line.

For example, if your 16-month-old baby typically has three nursing sessions per 24-hour period, try to cut it down to two. Once you're down to two, try cutting it down to one. Once you're down to one nursing session, try to skip it one day by going out when it normally occurs. Then, a few days later, try to skip that last remaining nursing session for two days in a row.

You can continue this gradual process until the day you can't quite recall when the last nursing session occurred.

For a *minority* of babies, cold-turkey weaning works at this age.

In contrast to the *majority* of babies, for whom a gradual weaning approach works best, for a *minority* of babies, cold-turkey weaning is an option after 16 months.

The babies who are easy to wean cold turkey at this age are those for whom breastfeeding no longer "works." Here's one example of breastfeeding "not working:" Your toddler fusses and you nurse him, and he stops fussing while he's latched on, but then the moment you stop nursing he starts fussing again. In this scenario, you feel like you've gained nothing by nursing.

Another example: you nurse your toddler down for naptime or nighttime, and then he's still awake. Awake, and clamouring for a

---

44 In some cases, such as a medical emergency, an abrupt weaning is necessary, but that's a different type of scenario, because in that case you're not setting a goal to wean fully—you're just doing it, and getting it done. Pronto. For information about and support for an abrupt weaning, see the breastfeeding resources listed at the end of this book.

back rub or a book. Again, in this scenario you feel like you've gained nothing by including breastfeeding in your bedtime routine.

In other words, weaning cold turkey may be the best approach in those cases where the breastfeeding ceases to be a handy tool for making momma's life easier.

Weaning cold turkey doesn't need much explanation: you just stop nursing. Full stop.

But two approaches to consider are a "vacation weaning" or "holiday weaning." Vacation weaning can happen when mom and baby are together but in a new environment, or when mom or baby goes on vacation without the other. Holiday weaning is possible when you have a special occasion with a bunch of visiting family members or house guests to distract baby. Basically, look for an opportunity when the normal routine gets turned upside down. For the minority of toddlers who are no longer relying on breastfeeding for soothing, a vacation or holiday environment will likely be distracting enough that they won't even notice that the nighttime ritual suddenly involves going straight from book time in the armchair to a belly-rub in the crib, with no breastfeeding in-between.

It helps to know that cold-turkey weaning after the age of 16 months normally **involves little to no crying**—if it's the right fit for your toddler. So, if you try to wean cold turkey and your baby gets upset, consider that you may need to change your mind, ditch the cold-turkey approach, and go back to gradual weaning.

Benefits to nursing a toddler

While there's no pressure to continue nursing at the 16- to 24-month stage if you feel done with it, there are still benefits to breastfeeding if you're not in a rush to wean:

- ✓ It's a great nap-starter for some toddlers.
- ✓ A great source of nutrition.
- ✓ A stuffed up, feverish, or sick toddler will often be willing to nurse even if he's rejecting other food and drink.

- ✓ Toddlers who breastfeed get an immune boost for fighting colds and other ailments, and so do nursing moms. This is handy if your toddler has just started daycare and you can't afford too many sick days at a time when it feels like your career has already taken a beating.

- ✓ Every additional month of breastfeeding decreases mom's lifetime risk of developing breast cancer.

- ✓ Helps baby's final jaw formation and reduces (but doesn't entirely eliminate) the likelihood of needing expensive orthodontics later in life. This means that when the dentist looks into your child's mouth when his baby teeth start falling out, she's more likely to say, "Oh yes, there's plenty of room for his adult teeth to come in." The active sucking motion that a toddler uses to nurse from the breast helps promote normal jaw widening (which is much, much cheaper than having an orthodontist take care of the jaw widening).

Bottom line: You're in charge at this stage. Wean if you want to wean. Breastfeed if you want to breastfeed.

Keep offering your toddler food and drink.

Your baby should be up to three or four larger meals per day at this stage, with a snack or two in between, for a total of four to six sittings at the table per day.

If it seems like your child hardly touched his food during some of these meals, that's okay. Don't worry about it. Clear away the plates. Mealtime is done. Babies and toddlers tend to meet their nutritional needs over the course of a week in irregularly sized meals—at times exhibiting a ravenous appetite and at other times just pecking a few bites.

You can also offer your child water in a cup several times each day. If he hasn't done so already, your toddler will soon fully master how to drink from an open cup without spilling its contents. He'll let you know when he's ready by pushing your helping hands away. "I do it!"

Keep putting your toddler down for his afternoon nap.

There are a few major sleep developments at this age.

First, the afternoon nap remains crucial.

The afternoon nap is still very important at this stage. The majority of babies drop the *morning* nap by 24 months, but it's too early to drop the *afternoon* nap. Health professionals say that children have a physiological need for at least one midday nap until about the age of three.

Second, be aware that many children stage a nap strike around this age—this doesn't mean they've outgrown the nap.

Some children begin (temporarily) refusing to go down for their afternoon nap **between about 20 and 24 months of age**. If your toddler falls into this category, it's because he's getting better at asserting his wants. And he *wants* to hang out with you! But wants and needs are two different things. Your baby's brain *needs* the rest. At this age your child has the capacity to stay awake all day, but that doesn't mean it's healthy for him, or that he should.

If you have a one-year-old baby who's hit the not-uncommon developmental milestone of suddenly resisting his last remaining nap, consider leaving him in his crib sobbing for at least **20 minutes** before you go back to soothe him to sleep a second time. Trying to soothe him back to sleep—rather than just picking him up at the 20-minute mark and carrying on with your day—is important because he still really needs that nap. If he doesn't fall asleep after the second soothing-to-sleep routine, then leave him crying for at least 20 minutes again. After that, consider a third attempt at soothing him to sleep, as long as the total time he spends crying in his crib (with intermittent soothing) doesn't exceed **one hour**.

This crying-before-the-nap isn't quite the same as sleep-training, because your baby has already learned the skill of falling into a deep sleep on his own. Rather, it's about sleep guarding.

Remember how I said in the previous chapter that when baby is ready to drop his morning nap you should go pick him up after 10 minutes of crying? Well, when it comes to a temporary strike that affects your child's last remaining daytime nap, a different guideline applies. It's in your baby's best interest that you power through and insist that the afternoon nap continue.

Nap strikes rarely last more than a few days to a week, so this crying is not your new normal. It's just a hiccup that you need to deal with.

An "afternoon nap strike" before 24 months is a bit like a "nursing strike" before 12 months—baby is simply too young to drop it, so momma needs to ride it out and do what it takes to get baby back on track.

One more tip: Baby's last remaining daytime nap should ideally be in the middle of the day, so that there's a roughly equivalent distribution of wakefulness before and after. If baby is resisting the afternoon nap, move it so it begins earlier in the day. If baby is resisting the nap at 1 pm, for example, try offering it at noon the next day. If baby resists at noon, try 11:30 am the next time.

Third: Bedtime resistance at night is also normal at this age.

Your little baby isn't so little anymore. He's turning into his own person, with growing awareness of everything. One of the things he's aware of is that everything *fun* happens *after* you've put him to bed. *Everything.* He'd be bananas to go to sleep just when the party's getting started! He positively, absolutely, no way, will not go to bed!

Be strong, because there's literally only one way to get through this stage with a reasonable bedtime intact.

Tears.

Baby's, for sure, and maybe yours.

When your toddler exhibits bedtime resistance, go through your usual routine, then tell him clearly that it's bedtime now and you will have to put him in his crib and leave. Then do just that—leave—and listen to him sobbing in his crib. He'll get tuckered out with all this protesting, so after 10 minutes go in for another round of soothing.

He'll likely be more open to it the second time. If not, leave him to cry for another 10 or 20 minutes, then move to round three of your bedtime soothing routine.

You're not trying to make your toddler cry himself to sleep—after all, you're well past the sleep-training period. What you're doing is resolutely safeguarding his sleep. You're also giving him a chance to express his emotions in a safe environment. *How dare you put me to bed when the adults are staying up?! I want to stay up with you! Come back here, you cotton-headed ninny muggins! I'm mad, mad, mad!*

Human beings need to express both positive and negative emotions. Instead of trying to suppress negative feelings, we should let our children know that it's okay to experience emotional ups and downs, that there's no need for them to hide their true feelings from the people they love. If your toddler has strong feelings about being sent to bed, it's okay for him to let the whole household know he's upset.

After he's let off steam for about 10 minutes on his own in a dark room (the kind of environment that will help him get into sleepytime mode), go back in and lovingly soothe him into sleep again. Once he's had a good cry, he may be more amenable to bedtime.

At this age your toddler's body needs to begin nighttime sleep as soon after 6:30 pm as possible. His protest is not a sign that he's ready to stay up late every night. His protest is a sign that he's becoming a vocal advocate for himself.

Remember: You're the parent, and you know that his best chance at a calm and happy toddlerhood comes from adequate nighttime rest. Bubby needs his sleep.

Fourth: Rest assured this doesn't mean endless wailing with every sleep.

What will change is the amount of crying. Between about four months to about 20 months of age, a sleep-trained baby will fall asleep with no tears most days and a few light tears on rare days. Sometime after about 20 months, however, the scenario flips and you may enter a **temporary** period where, on most days, you can expect about two to ten minutes of crying at bedtime, while on *rare* days your baby will go down with no tears at all.

When this happens, parents are sometimes tempted to push bedtime back with the hope that a more tired baby will be ready to sleep without tears. Alas, all you'll end up with is a more tired baby! A 6:30 pm bedtime is still best for this age group.

This two-to-ten-minutes-of-protest-crying at bedtime is, again, not a sign that bedtime has suddenly become a problem. Rather, it's a sign that your toddler is now aware that he'd much rather stay up with you. Your choice, as parent, is to either give in to baby's desire to stay up late and deal with on-and-off elevated crankiness all day tomorrow, or, take a deep breath and accept ten minutes of crying tonight. He's simply expressing how he feels.

And take heart. In a few weeks—you probably won't even notice when—he'll go back to falling asleep with no tears on most days and a few light tears on rare days.

There's a bonus to allowing your developing child to express his feelings about bedtime.

Every time your child recovers and feels okay again after a difficult emotion, he becomes a little more resilient. One of your jobs as a parent is to support your child as he learns to deal with strong feelings—not to prevent those feelings from happening or plowing them out of the way when they do.

To be emotionally equipped for a healthy adulthood, a human being needs to start out with child-sized experiences of making do with the hand he's been dealt. The old parenting trope—"You get what you get, and you don't get upset"—sets us up for a stoic existentialism:

> Know you are doomed.
> Accept the pointlessness of existence.
> Enjoy yourself anyway.

Finally, be aware that a well-rested toddler generally wakes up happy.

Once he wakes up, he'll rouse slowly and start babbling to his stuffies and imaginary friends. The babbling is important because it tells you he got the sleep he needed. Fetch your toddler from his crib as soon as possible after the contented babbling begins—you want to reassure him that you're not going to leave him waiting for you when he's in awake mode.

> **Pro tip:**
>
> Experienced parents know that a baby monitor needs to be used judiciously. So, don't turn on the monitor until after baby has fallen asleep. If he's crying at bedtime, there's no need to amplify the sound. You can already hear him perfectly well! But if you turn it on once he's soundly asleep, you'll be able to hear his gentle murmurs and stirrings as soon he wakes up, so you can pick him up from his crib promptly.

If your one-year-old baby wakes up crying, however, then either something in his environment woke him up before he was ready, or you missed the contented-babbling stage and he's wondering where you are. If there is crying at the end of a nap or bedtime, it's a sign that mom and dad need to do some problem solving; something needs to be fixed. A well-rested toddler normally wakes up happy.

It's time to teach your toddler how to use playground equipment.

Ah, I'm just messing with you again.
Listen, one day your child will need you to teach him how to tie his shoelaces. He will need you to teach him how to drive. There are plenty of skills that require your help.

But your toddler does not need you to explain how to use playground equipment.

Playgrounds are designed by highly paid (I assume) playground designers to be used (and figured out) by children. Consider this: Your clever little toddler might just know a thing or two more than you do about how the playground equipment is meant to be used. He doesn't need you to dish out a running coach's commentary at the park.

And yet when you're at your local park, you'll find plenty of adults who step in thinking they know more about playground equipment than their kids:

"On your bum, Emma! Good girl!"

"Hold onto the railing, Grayson! Good boy!"

"Nuh, uh, don't touch the ladder, Charlotte!"

Or that perennial favourite: "Don't climb up the slide!" (Slides are actually designed to be used in both directions—a feature that is delightfully obvious to children. It's why the slide sides have that rounded little lip for gripping.)

So here's a parent-tested tip to get the most out of your next visit to the playground or local green space: See how long you can go without dishing out a single instruction to your newly mobile toddler. I'll bet, if you try really hard, you can last the whole visit without issuing a single rule or directive. Your toddler—the one who managed to figure out crawling and walking—is expertly qualified for this task. He was born to move and explore.

And here's another tip for your time at the park: There's no need to follow your toddler in lockstep or stay within arm's reach. "Stay within arm's reach" is the safety requirement for swimming pools, not toddler-friendly parks and houses.

If you stay within arm's reach at the playground, you'll be tempted to play with your child at the playground, and that's a risky proposition for both of you. Playing isn't the problem. Playing is good! The bad idea is joining in on the playtime: when adults do it, it always seems stilted and unnatural: "Hey, let's pretend to be horsies! Wheee!"

Inevitably, you'll end up doing the restless, lockstep, zombie shuffle one sees so often at the park these days, with the shadowed child looking bewildered and the adult looking zoned out ("Mmm, hmm...") or pouring out the treacly goo of unnecessarily upbeat enthusiasm ("Good job, Henry!").[45]

It isn't easy to step back from active parenting after the first year of holding our babies close and being involved with every single aspect of their day.

You need to be like the British royals when it comes to government affairs—observing but not meddling. As Queen Mary advises her granddaughter, Queen Elizabeth II, in an episode of *The Crown*, "To do nothing is the hardest job of all. And it will take every ounce of energy that you have." It truly will.

If he runs, resist chasing him.

If he's doing something new, be mindful of whether you actually need to say, "No, you can't."

If he's trying to climb, don't help him up.

Case in point: If you lift up your toddler to the top of the slide platform, he'll have no sense of how high he is or how dangerous it would be to step through one of the openings. Instead, stand back and let him figure it out. Shortly after his first birthday, your baby may figure out how to get up on the first rung of the tot ladder. In all likelihood, he'll then fall through between the rungs, into a bed of pea gravel or some other safety surface that can cushion his impact from such a short falling distance. And now he's learned something about his body and his surroundings. If you don't rush in to save him, he'll figure out how to safely get on the first rung of the ladder and he won't get to the second one until he's ready.

---

[45] Here's where peer pressure comes in. If there are five caregivers at the local park, and you're the only one who's not within arm's reach of a newly mobile baby, I'm not gonna sugarcoat this: you'll feel awkward about it. On the one hand, you don't want peer pressure and the fear of looking like a negligent parent to compromise your approach. On the other hand, it's not like anyone wants to hear you lecture them about helicopter parenting. No one appointed you sheriff of this playground. So, if you're not lucky enough to have other like-minded parents at the park with you, then you may end up sitting all alone in your camping chair at the periphery, looking like a hoser. Hang in there. Hopefully, with enough visits to the playground, you'll eventually meet "your people," who'll bring their own camping chairs, and maybe a few beers, and join you.

The playground is a great place for small children to practise making these sorts of small mistakes, because playgrounds are designed to keep children as safe *as necessary*. Practising making judgment calls when the stakes are low makes a person better at making judgment calls in the future, when the stakes are high.

By the time he's figured out, on his own, how to get all the way up to the platform at the top of the slide, he'll have enough experience under his belt to know that plunging off the edge would hurt.

Another danger with lifting your baby to the top of the slide: you risk interfering with the normal, healthy development of his muscle strength. Fitness isn't just about the absence of obesity. It's also about acquiring the minimum strength and basic movement skills required to enjoy sports and take part in other activities that require vigour and coordination.

Numerous studies have found that strength and fitness levels are declining among children. Compared to previous generations, there are increasing numbers of "wet noodles:" kids who struggle to lift their feet up to their hands while gripping monkey bars at age three, kick a soccer ball at age four, climb 20 feet up a tree at age five, or complete a 40 km bike ride at age six (none of which are remarkable feats).

Muscle weakness isn't something that toddlers just outgrow. Health experts have noticed that weak children become weak teenagers and weak teenagers become weak adults. Now is the best time to let your child figure out, on his own, how to get to the top of the slide, using whatever approach he chooses.

By the same token, if your toddler approaches a piece of playground equipment that he can't climb onto or use on his own, then it's too advanced for him and probably not safe for him to use. By standing back and letting him explore the parts of the playground that he can figure out on his own, you allow your toddler to experience his world at his own pace.

The irony is that, once your baby becomes mobile, you may be doing a lot of baby-wearing around the house, with your toddler held close; then, when you're out and about, you do a lot of letting go, with your toddler running free. It's not attachment parenting. It's not free-range parenting. It's a little bit of both.

Your child is looking for you to be both a presence and an absence as he grows.

CHAPTER 14:

Months 24 to 36

Welcome to the Toilet-Training Twos!

Age two is when most (not all—but most) toddlers transition from full-time diapers to full-time underwear. Keep in mind, though, that there are 12 whole months when your child is two. Toilet-training takes months to unfold; it's not a regimented exercise that takes two or three days to complete. You've got all year to work on this.

Start by introducing the theory.

For starters, if you haven't already done so, let your toddler have a peek at what happens in the bathroom, whenever the opportunity naturally presents itself. Simply leave the door open when it works for *you* and let him follow you in when it works for *him*.[46]

You can also begin introducing simple concepts, such as:

---

[46] As an aside, it makes it easier on everyone if boys sit when they first learn how to pee on a toilet. There's less mess and there are fewer concepts to learn, because they'll follow the same steps for poo and for pee.
And don't worry—no one will have to teach your son how to pee standing up later on. He'll have magically figured that out on his own by the time he starts kindergarten, without any instructions from you.

"I've really gotta go! I'm going to run, run, run to the toilet!"
"Mommy is wearing underwear!"
"Mommy does not have a diaper!"
"Pee pee and poo poo do NOT go in Mommy's underwear."
"Pee pee goes in the toilet."
"Mommy is done. Mommy's going to flush."
"Bye-bye pee pee, bye-bye poo poo!"

It's no big deal—we sit on the toilet. It's just something we do around here.

Book *Toilet-Training Days!* into your calendar.

Here is where things really start to come together.

With toilet-training, the conventional wisdom is to wait until a child is "ready." This makes perfect sense, except one thing: How on earth is a parent supposed to *know* when a child is ready?

Many families find that pre-scheduling *Toilet-Training Days* is a technique that bridges this gap. Pre-scheduling the training makes your life easier because it gives your baby semi-regular opportunities to practise all the skills involved in using a toilet—and, as we all know, practice makes perfect! And it provides parents with a stress-free, tear-free, gentle way of determining when their toddler is "ready."

Okay, so here's what you do: When your toddler reaches his second birthday, bring up your calendar and find a day every month, or month and a half, when you can devote the morning to toilet-training. You're looking to block off about eight to 12 days between when your child is 24 and 36 months old. Make sure it's clearly blocked off: **Toilet-Training Day!** Hold that spot in your agenda the way you would any other important appointment. The days don't have to be evenly spaced out. It may be that with your busy schedule you'll end up scheduling Toilet-Training Days two weeks in a row followed by a gap of a couple of months. That's fine. Feel free to work around all the other things you have going on in your life.

The purpose of your pre-scheduled *Toilet-Training Days* is not to achieve success, but rather to practise failure.

This is key, so let's hear it again, once more with feeling! *The purpose of Toilet-Training Days is not to achieve success, but instead to literally— and I'm serious about this—practise failure.* The *Toilet-Training Days* provide a semi-regular opportunity for your baby to slowly practise all the new concepts and skills he needs to learn, without any expectation that he will transition from diapers to underwear.

This is also why the first *Toilet-Training Day* should be scheduled when your baby is as close to 24 months as possible. The vast majority of babies aren't yet ready to fully toilet-train at that age, but all regularly developing children are definitely old enough to begin practising the skills involved. If you wait too long you risk missing the developmental window where it all comes together, easy as pie— meaning you'll still be able to toilet-train, but it'll be a lot more work.

For about the first half of the year, it helps to keep the *Toilet-Training Day* relatively short.

You just need a few hours, about once every month or so.

For the first few sessions, begin the training after breakfast ends (or maybe right after you've changed the morning poopy diaper) and wrap things up before lunchtime. In other words, the "day" ends up being more like a couple of hours. Once your child is back in his diaper, you won't need to do any more practising until the next date comes up in your calendar.

When your toddler is around two-and-a-half, however, you may want to ramp things up. Consider starting the underwear time before breakfast and continuing with it through lunch, before returning him to a diaper for his afternoon nap.

Hydrate.

Offer your toddler lots of water, to encourage frequent elimination. Juice isn't normally recommended for children, but consider offering it on a *Toilet-Training Day.* The sugary goodness will encourage your toddler to guzzle it down, which will in turn encourage him to pee more often.

No pullups.

This should almost go without saying, but pull-ups defeat the purpose and prolong the process.

Clear your schedule.

You can't multi-task on a *Toilet-Training Day.* No conference calls. No grocery runs. No returning emails. No dishwashing. You need to focus 100 percent on your little Schnookums.

> Okay, so you've got the *Toilet-Training Days* in your calendar? Great!
> Now we wait for the first one to arrive…

All right, it's a *Toilet-Training Day!*

First, let your toddler know the plan. "Today we're going to practise using the toilet!"

Then take off your toddler's diaper and help him put on his underwear and pants. Don't change his clothes in the bathroom, because running *to* the bathroom is one of the skills you're going to practise this morning. "These are dry pants. This is dry underwear. Look. There's no pee pee in your underwear. Look. There is no poo poo in your underwear. Pee pee and poo poo go in the toilet. Let's practise!"

Then help him run to the bathroom, pull off his pants and underwear, and sit on the toilet. Then pretend to wipe, pretend to flush, put his clothes back on, and wash up.

Some kids are okay with sitting on the toilet for a bit, but the majority just want to bounce right back up and go on to the next step. For the most part, don't bother trying to convince your toddler to spend more time on the toilet than he wants to. At this stage, there's nothing to be gained by continuing to sit on the toilet until pee comes out, because then he'll miss out on the lesson of what an accident feels like.

Many toddlers will be thrilled to spend the morning running back and forth to the toilet, practising. If you've seen the *Karate Kid* movies, you'll feel like the title character by the end of the day, repeating the same motions over and over and over. ("Wax on/Wax off" in the classic 1984 version starring Ralph Macchio, and "Jacket on/Jacket off" in the equally delightful 2010 version with Jaden Smith.)

But if your toddler is fully unimpressed by the idea of toilet practice, don't worry. Let him just hang out in his underwear. There's no need to force the practising if he's done after the first go-round.

There are a few more concepts to practise, but first you need to wait until your toddler pees his pants. You *want* an accident, because the sensation of wet underwear will help your child learn about the difference between a diaper and underwear.

Once your child has an accident, you can help him understand what happened: "Oh no! You pee peed in your pants. Now your pants are wet. Wet is *yucky*."

Be matter-of-fact about this, rather than harsh. You're trying to relay useful information, not discipline your child. Your child hasn't done anything wrong, and you're not trying to fix his behaviour. You're just informing him that pee pee feels worse in underwear than it does in a diaper.

"Let's practise again!" Once you have your child changed into a fresh, dry pair of underwear and pants, you can run him through the steps of how to use the toilet again.

One aspect many parents appreciate about pre-scheduled *Toilet-Training Days* is that there are many opportunities for positive reinforcement. Most children never pee or poo into the potty even once during the pre-scheduled *Toilet-Training Days*, but you'll be able to check your toddler's underwear for dryness periodically and say, "Oh, your underwear is still dry! That's wonderful! Dry underwear feels good!"

But the **best** part of pre-booking a *Toilet-Training Day* is that once the scheduled practice time is over, it's over. Back to diapers!

Your toddler has likely never done anything this complex before. Between holding it in and pulling off pants and flushing there are around two dozen steps involved—only one of which involves getting pee into the toilet. This is why it helps to pre-schedule these practise sessions. If your toddler has committed the motions to memory by the time his body is physiologically ready, then the transition to wearing underwear full time will be smoother.

This is the easiest, most stress-free way to toilet-train your toddler. No one single *Toilet-Training Day* is meant to be *it*—the day your child is fully toilet-trained. Instead, every *Toilet-Training Day* will simply be a chance to hang out and help junior practise the skills he'll need one day in the future.

And guess what—one magical *Toilet-Training Day*—when he's ready, it will all suddenly click and, just like that—he'll be toilet-trained! But he's the expert of his own body. He'll let you know when you've reached the last *Toilet-Training Day.* And if that last one doesn't take place until sometime when he's three or four, no problem. Every child hits developmental milestones at a different rate. When they're 10, no one will know—or care—which kid figured out the toilet at 19 months and which kid did it at age three.

The goal isn't for your child to use the toilet. The goal is for your child to have dry underwear.

If you use this as a measure of success, it'll be much easier to know when your child has figured it out. The *Toilet-Training Days* you've scheduled in your calendar *aren't* over when your child finally figures out that pee or poo goes in the toilet. You'll still need to put your child back in diapers at the end of those training days. Rather, *Toilet-Training Days* will be done one magical day when your child goes through the whole morning with dry underwear, and then through lunch and naptime and beyond, and voilà! Dry underwear! All day!

This doesn't mean your child will never again have an accident, of course, once you've gone through your first full day with dry underwear, but pee or poo in the underwear needs to be an *exceptional* occurrence once you move on from full-time diapers. If you're dealing with frequently soiled underwear, everyone will be a lot less stressed if junior just goes back to wearing absorbent disposables for a few more weeks or months and then tries again on the next *Toilet Training Day.*

You can do this. Your toddler can do this.

This approach to toilet training is based on what moms have shared at my workshops, and the good news is that it's easier than you think. Soon you'll be able to toss those dirty diapers for good!

Speaking of transitions, it's time to kick weaning into high gear.

Breastfeeding is age-appropriate for a two-year-old child.

If no one you know is nursing a toddler, keep in mind that plenty of two-year-olds are using soothers, sucking their thumbs, and bottle-feeding to sleep, all of which satisfy their need for touch and security. Breastfeeding is directly related to these other three methods of oral soothing, but with the added bonus of giving your child nutrition, boosting his immune responses, and contributing to the healthier development of his teeth and jaws.

This is why breastfeeding is age-appropriate and beneficial for a two-year-old child.

But let's call out the elephant in the room.

Moms can feel like they deserve accolades for figuring out how to nurse their newborns—"breast is best" and all that. Then, to top it off, the World Health Organization vaguely allows that breastfeeding "may continue for two years or more." So far, so good...And yet, despite official sanctions, moms who are nursing toddlers are well aware that they've crossed the line from doing something that enjoys widespread societal approval to doing something that seems vaguely eccentric. It can feel complicated, when it shouldn't.

It's really very simple:

- It's perfectly natural and normal to nurse a two-year-old child at your breast. If you and your child aren't done with nursing at this age, you go ahead and nurse.
- By the same token, though, you don't get bonus momma points for breastfeeding your two-year-old. So if you're done with nursing at this age, go ahead and wean your toddler.

In other words, breastfeeding your two-year-old is totally your call: Do it if it works for you and don't do it if it doesn't.

Active, momma-led weaning is a good idea at this age.

But here's the catch: regardless of whether you're a fully-happy-and-confident breastfeeding momma (rock it, girl!) or a fully-completely-ready-to-wean momma (you rock it, too!), age two is when you ***need*** to introduce weaning practices into your bag of tricks, if you haven't yet done so.

Now, if you're a happy nursing momma you may be wondering why it's necessary to introduce weaning practices. Answer: Weaning *practices* are not the same thing as actual, completed weaning. Even if you're not ready to fully wean yet, you *will* be ready to fully wean at some point, and the weaning practices you introduce now will make things go a whole lot smoother when that time comes.

Some speak of the holy grail of a "natural weaning." Let me tell you: There's no such thing. If you nurse your toddler with the same unabashed enthusiasm as a newborn baby, then one terrible, horrible day you or your child will be ready to wean before the other is ready, and there will be tears—oh yes, from both of you—and nails-sliding-on-chalkboard irritation, and angst, and anxiety and gloom. You don't want that.

Because it's easier on everyone when breastfeeding phases out on a happy note, if you haven't yet done so then now is the time to introduce one or more weaning practices into your daily routine (you'll find concrete suggestions for this in the previous two chapters).

Nursing less than once per day

A huge milestone, once you get there, is going your first full day without nursing. When you're down to that last nursing, not having it happen every day feels inconceivable, but with a bit of planning (like momma being out of the house at the given time), you can get a child down to nursing every second day or less, which brings you that much closer to full weaning. Try to arrange a few days per month—and then a few days per week—where you're not around at the time when that last-to-go nursing session still tends to happen, so that someone else has to meet your child's need for soothing.

Some toddlers are easier to wean than others.

Some toddlers just have a naturally stronger oral fixation. If you have a hard-to-wean toddler, then this is the same kid who would likely be struggling with a seemingly unbreakable thumb-sucking or soother-using habit at this age (and who may very well be demanding a thumb and a soother *in addition to* breastfeeding!).

It's about the journey, not the destination.

If you and your little pumpkin treasure the nursing relationship you have right now, remember that introducing weaning practices doesn't mean that you are weaning *fully*. You're just *weaning*. It's an active verb. You need to leave the start line, even if you don't intend to hit the finish line just yet.

Keep offering your toddler healthy food and drink choices.

Your toddler is a bear with very little brain. You can't reason with him. So, if you don't want him to harass you for candy, cookies, crackers, granola bars, pop, chocolate milk, potato chips, juice, or gummy bears, then never offer him any candy, cookies, crackers, granola bars, pop, chocolate milk, potato chips, or gummy bears—not at this age, anyway.

Save some of the good stuff for the preschool years when his cognitive skills have developed enough that you can plan, negotiate, and delay treat times. Toddlers are too young for beer; that's an adult privilege. They're also too young for sugary treats; that's a preschooler privilege.

Some people claim that if you offer children both healthy and unhealthy options, they'll satisfy their craving for sugary and salty snacks and then naturally gravitate to the healthy choices. That's what *some* people claim. Most mommas will tell you that's utter malarkey. Ask parents who've let their kids have the run of the beautiful buffet at an all-inclusive beach resort—by the end of a one-week stay, children of any age will be reaching for nothing but white buns and chocolate ice cream. Your kids won't make healthy choices unless you eliminate the unhealthy options.

Continue to put your toddler down for his afternoon nap.

The afternoon nap continues to be very important.

All children need to keep the single nap until around the age of three, and some children continue napping until age six.

By the age of two, children are better at handling the occasional skipped afternoon nap during a vacation or fun family outing. Let your toddler skip the afternoon nap too many days in a row, though, and you'll end up with a two-year-old who has frequent temper tantrums and total meltdowns. Naptime is still crucial for your toddler's brain development and emotional regulation.

Nap length

Some children shorten their naps at this age; you may find the three-hour afternoon nap has turned into a two-hour siesta. Other children continue full speed with a long nap until they're ready to drop it cold turkey. It's usually best to let your two-year-old decide how long naptime should last.

The afternoon nap does not interfere with bedtime.

When their toddler or preschooler is having a hard time with his evening bedtime, parents sometimes misinterpret this as a sign that it's time to drop the afternoon nap.

However, if a tricky bedtime is the problem you're trying to solve, eliminating the afternoon nap isn't the solution. Instead, consider moving naptime to an earlier start. Maybe you need to serve lunch at 11 am and start the afternoon nap shortly before noon.

Contrary to common but misguided opinion, it's not the *presence* of an afternoon nap that interferes with night sleep. It is the *absence* of the afternoon nap that interferes with night sleep.

Around this age, children drop their last nap.

Around age three (earlier for some children and later for others), kids will transition from one nap per day to no nap. Of all the nap eliminations, this one is the lengthiest—for some kids it can take several months to complete.

Some transitions require heavy parental intervention while others occur naturally. Dropping the afternoon nap—as you might have guessed—is fully child-led.

That being said, if your two-year-old is under 30 months, a refusal to nap is unlikely to be a reflection of developmental readiness to fully phase out the afternoon nap. Something else is likely interrupting your child's needed sleep time, so you need to do everything in your power to get the nap back on track.

After around 30 months, on the other hand, a refusal to nap is likely an indication that your child is developmentally ready to power through most days without sleeping.

Remember how toddlers are prone to temporary nap strikes around 20 months of age, and that the solution is to leave your child in his crib—even if he's crying—for at least 20 to 60 minutes before you go get him?

After about 30 months of age, if your preschooler resists going down for a nap, then only leave him protesting, fussing, or crying in his bed for about 10 or 15 minutes. After that, just go get him and soothe away his tears. He's not going to fall asleep this afternoon.

This could just be a one-off occurrence, but if you start to notice that you have more than one episode in one week where he doesn't fall asleep easily, then you officially have a child who is beginning to transition away from an afternoon nap.

A preschooler who no longer naps still needs his nap routine.

Because the loss of the afternoon nap happens quite slowly, what you'll find is that, instead of dropping it cold turkey, your preschooler will nap four to five days per week for a few weeks, and then three to four days per week for a few weeks, and then two to three days per week for a few weeks, and so on.

The challenge is that you won't know which days *are* the napping days and which ones *aren't*.

To support your child with this difficult transition, make sure you incorporate *quiet time* into each afternoon.[47] From now on, instead of soothing your child down to an afternoon nap, your job will be to soothe your child to afternoon quiet time, and then leave it up to him whether he wants to fall asleep.

That reminds me: this is also the point at which your child is ideally suited to transitioning from a crib to a regular bed, if he hasn't already done so. A bed will make it easier for him to leave his sleeping area any time he likes.

A key point to this new routine of afternoon quiet time is that if your toddler starts fussing or crying in his room—the room that he is perfectly capable of leaving, by the way, because he's not in a crib and his door is ajar—don't rush in too quickly. Give him a bit of

---

47 If your child is attending a childcare program, the daycare will likely have an afternoon naptime for everybody. Even if your child has dropped the afternoon nap at home, it's important to support the nap routine at daycare. Children get tuckered out by all the goings-on at childcare centres, which make them more inclined to fall asleep. And even if your child doesn't fall asleep, the quiet provides a needed time-out for his little brain.

time—maybe ten minutes or so—in case he's trying to work his way into a nap.

Here are two examples of how afternoon quiet time might turn out on any given day.

Scenario #1: Your child *doesn't* fall asleep after the routine.

You cheerfully declare, "It's quiet time!" You head to the bedroom, you draw the curtains closed, you snuggle together in his big bed, and you read two or three naptime stories. Then you say, "Sweet dreams…Bye, bye!"

Instead of closing the door to the bedroom, you leave it slightly ajar, so your child can leave the room if he chooses.

What happens next depends on your child. Perhaps he'll engage in 40 minutes of babbling conversation with the stuffies on his bed. Perhaps he'll ramp up from babbling to fussing and calls for momma. And perhaps after 10 minutes of fussing (not quite crying) that's slowly ramping up, you come and get him and say, "Hello! Quiet time is over for today!"

In this example, your toddler did not sleep, but he still managed to get some rest for his brain during the downtime.

And momma got almost an hour to herself!

Scenario #2: Your child *does* fall asleep after the naptime routine.

Same bedtime routine, but this time after 40 minutes of babbling conversation with the stuffies on his bed, your baby starts fussing and calling for momma, and after 10 minutes you start heading for the stairs, when you stop midway and notice…*silence.* Your preschooler has unexpectedly fallen asleep.

This is a minor change to be aware of. For most of the past couple of years, your child likely fell asleep for his afternoon nap within about five or ten minutes of you leaving the room, and almost never with any fussing or crying. After about 30 months of age, your child is likely to be awake for much longer before falling asleep, and on those rare days when he does nap, it's more likely to be preceded by fussing or light crying.

Explaining pre-nap tears

Some parents may struggle with the pre-nap fussing or crying that suddenly starts at this age and mistake it for a sign that their child no longer needs a nap at all, or that their child's nighttime sleep is negatively affected by the daytime nap.

That is not the case.

There are plenty of times when our minds *want* one thing and our bodies *need* another thing. You know how an evening glass of wine or two with friends makes you feel good, and the evening is winding down, and your mind thinks, "Oh, I could totally go for one more glass of wine right now," but you know your body (your liver, your love handles, your ability to function at work tomorrow) does *not* need one more glass of wine right now. Your body says, "Be happy with the two glasses of wine you already had!"

That's how you need to interpret your toddler's pre-sleep fussing.

His mind is saying, "Oh, I could totally go for some more play time right now. My body won't mind if we have just one more hour of awake time. Just *one* more. It'll feel so *gooood*," while his body is saying, "Sleep! Go to sleep!"

Continuing this new quiet-time routine well past the time when your child starts dropping the afternoon nap provides him with the best opportunity for catching some zzz's when his body needs them.

Even if your child doesn't fall asleep, afternoon quiet time in his bed is crucial because, once they drop the regular nap, children are still in the phase where **one** nap is too many, but "**none** is not enough." So they get cranky. Afternoon quiet time helps take the edge off that crankiness.

And remember, with his bedroom door ajar, he can leave any time he likes. You're not forcing your baby to nap. You're just setting him up with a nap opportunity. (A napportunity!?)

New development: later bedtime at night.

Many families find bedtime starts to creep closer to 7 pm around the time their child turns two. It gets harder and harder to stick to the old 6:30 pm bedtime.

Then, after about 30 months, or around the same time as they drop their afternoon nap, many preschoolers move bedtime again, to around 7:30 pm. Preschool-aged human beings who don't get an afternoon nap seem biologically wired to stay up just a little bit later; it seems counter-intuitive, but that's just the way it works.

Once your baby's bedtime moves to 7:30 pm, it will likely stay there for a few years.

If night-waking resumes, get creative.

The steps involved in caring for a newborn baby are almost universal. A one-size-fits-most approach will work just fine in the vast majority of cases. But with every passing day, individual differences emerge, and by the time children are two years old, a one-size-fits-most approach becomes harder and harder to apply, including with breastfeeding. For example:

> Should you breastfeed your 30-month-old?
>
> I don't know. What do *you* think you should do, Momma?

Addressing the night-waking that will occasionally occur (as it does for all humans of any age) is another area that becomes more complicated at this age.

Your toddler may be up tonight for all sorts of reasons. For example, fears are common between the ages of two and four. Your child—the same child who's been sleeping soundly through the night for years—may now start waking up because of nightmares or scary sounds. Or maybe his blanket slid off and now he's chilly. Or maybe he's stuffed up from a cold. Or maybe, or maybe, who knows?

So, if your two-year-old has unexpectedly started a night-waking habit, how do you fix it tonight?

I don't know.

As a first step, go with your gut. What do *you* think you should do to get your toddler to stop night-waking tonight?

If your gut isn't giving you any winning suggestions, then ask your friends for ideas.

If your friends are coming up short, then ask the internet for uninformed speculation.

Or how about gentle, no-cry solutions? I know I mocked these earlier at the night-weaning and sleep-training stages, but your child is now at an age when gentle, no-cry nighttime solutions are called for. Perhaps a night-light will help? Perhaps you could leave the bedroom door ajar? Perhaps you need to make a big show of catching all the "monsters" at bedtime? Perhaps you don't mind getting up once or more per night to soothe your child in his own bed with some nighttime cuddles?

Or perhaps you're okay with letting him come into the family bed in the middle of the night, even if you haven't been co-sleeping before now?

Trying to resolve night-waking after 24 months is much trickier than it was at the infant stage. It takes some creativity.

If this all sounds a bit ambiguous as the step-by-step instructional part of this book draws to its end, that, happily, is the nature of parenting from here on in. The manual that came with your baby will get shelved. You won't need it any more.

Here they come: The last, lilting steps of the baby years.

Your baby is about to turn three! Plan a birthday party. Buy balloons, bake a cake, and invite all your favourite people to celebrate.

The baby years are coming to an end and you're heading into the fun and fascinating territory of the preschool years. I hope they bring your whole family more wonder, joy and, above all, love.

Love,

Susan

PART III:

TROUBLESHOOTING

CHAPTER 15:

Formula

> "What no one ever tells you about parenting is that every decision seems like the wrong one. You wander through life trying to make the least bad decisions for your kids, and watch your neighbours make different ones with a mixture of horror and envy."
>
> – Elizabeth Renzetti, *The Globe and Mail*,
> August 29, 2020

I've talked a lot about breastfeeding in this book, and perhaps you feel the approach has been a little one-sided. Well. In my defense, studies show that around 80 to 90 percent of women want to try breastfeeding when their babies are born. Majority rules! Breastfeeding is what most moms want help with.

Those same studies, however, show that only about 50 percent of moms are still breastfeeding when their babies are six months old. The other 30 to 40 percent intended to breastfeed, but stopped sooner than they planned. For myriad reasons, many women aren't meeting the breastfeeding goals they set for themselves. Women *want* to breastfeed, but don't always find it easy to do.

If you're nourishing your baby with formula—and it's your business whether that's by choice or by circumstance—I assume you'll figure out how to do it. You rarely hear of a mom failing to reach her bottlefeeding goal.

But data shows that moms need lots of accurate information and support to get breastmilk going. Winging it won't cut it.

So if you're a bottlefeeding momma, please know that I fully support the way you're nourishing your baby and please don't take offense at all the breastfeeding references. Just adjust them to fit your reality. When I say, "Nurse your baby to sleep," I know you'll figure out how to soothe your sweet pea to sleep in other ways.

Let's also put the risks of formula into perspective. The science is clear: formula increases health risks for baby, which is why health professionals recommend breastmilk. But for moms who aren't breastfeeding—and again, your reasons are your business—let's look at the bigger picture. It's true that by nourishing your baby with formula, you're increasing certain risk factors for him, but it's also true that every parent ends up making choices that increase risk factors for their children.

So maybe you're bottlefeeding formula. But maybe the serene breastfeeder sitting next to you is shorting her child on the sleep he needs for his brain development. Or maybe a few years down the road she could end up feeding her child a diet that exceeds daily recommended amounts of added sugar. Excessive screen time has its risks, too, yet society doesn't seem to agonize over screen time the way it does over formula. Jumpin' Jehoshaphat, there are a thousand and one ways to increase risks for our children; how we nourish them shortly after birth is just the tip of the iceberg. We're all—every single one of us—going to engage in parenting behaviours throughout our children's lives that increase risk.

Don't forget, too, that "increased risk" isn't a *guarantee* that something will go wrong. Smoking increases your risk of cancer, but it doesn't mean you'll get lung cancer. It just increases the probability. By the same token, *not* smoking doesn't guarantee you *won't* get lung cancer. Not smoking just decreases the probability.

And let's look at this whole "increased risk" business from another lens. (Yes, let's do that right after I very nearly made a direct link between formula and cigarettes.) Research shows that, over the *long term*, breastfeeding has comparatively *less* effect on a child's future health and IQ than other modifiable factors such as getting enough sleep, being surrounded by books, eating a well-balanced diet, and spending heaps of time on imaginative play.

And the long-term risks of formula fall away almost entirely when compared to the number one non-modifiable factor: the family you're born into. The social determinants of health exert a powerful influence on how we fare in life. If you and your partner are healthy, well educated, and can afford the home you live in, then there's a pretty good chance your baby will follow suit, regardless of whether he's breastfed.

That said, I don't want to sugarcoat facts and reassure you that formula is just as good as breastmilk. It isn't.

It's not as good as breastmilk. But it's good enough. And at the end of the day, that's all we can strive for with any aspect of our parenting.

Breastfeeding your baby is great, but ultimately, feeding your baby is the first priority. So if you are feeding your baby, give yourself a pat on the back!

Finding a supportive community is also important. A good place to start is googling "fearless formula feeder", but there are plenty of other ways to find virtual and actual communities of like-minded mothers out there.

Bottom line: You don't have to breastfeed to be a good mother. There are many wonderful moms who nourish and love with bottles.

CHAPTER 16:

Breastmilk

This chapter provides an overview of breastfeeding. It repeats the same information you'll find in the chronological, age-based chapters, but pulls all the breastfeeding tips into one chapter, so you can see the big picture of your nursing journey. Think of this as your breastfeeding cheat sheet: all the basics, in one spot.

Breastfeeding *is* possible. You can do it!

For hundreds of thousands of years, humans have fed their young with breastmilk. It's a basic evolutionary truth that our bodies are designed to breastfeed, so if your goal is to breastfeed, you should have every confidence that you *can* do it.

In the vast majority of cases, the number one factor that determines whether a mom can breastfeed isn't whether her body is physiologically capable of producing breastmilk (it most likely is), but whether she receives accurate information and support before baby arrives.

Like learning to talk and sing and love, breastfeeding is natural, but the guidance we receive from others makes a crucial difference in the learning process. Fred Rogers (star of *Mr. Rogers' Neighborhood*, an American children's TV show that ran for several decades in the late 20th century) once warmly observed that "…from the time you were very little, you've had people who have smiled you into smiling, people who have talked you into talking, sung you into singing, loved you into loving."

Some of our most basic human abilities are learned. So it's only natural that a new momma would need supportive people around to guide her into breastfeeding, too.

Health professionals recommend breastfeeding.

There are several reasons health professionals recommend that mothers breastfeed. But before I get into the good that comes from nursing, I wanted to dispel one pervasive myth: breastfeeding does not increase attachment.

What I mean is, breastfeeding is good for the parent-baby bond, sure, but you don't *need* to breastfeed to build attachment. Babies whose parents don't breastfeed still attach to their parents just fine.

So, if it's not a necessity for attachment, what is it good for?

For starters, *colostrum*, the early milk your body produces in the first few days after birth, is a highly concentrated superfood.

Colostrum doesn't just satisfy a newborn baby's thirst and hunger, it also protects against infections. And it's also effective at clearing meconium (your baby's first stools), which helps reduce jaundice.

Breastmilk is a low-cost, organic source of nutrition.

Formulas don't have all the nutritional elements found in breastmilk. They contain, for example, no antibodies, no enzymes, no living cells, no intestinal soothers, and no growth hormones. They contain much more aluminum, lead, cadmium, manganese, and iron than breastmilk. The proteins and fats in formula are also fundamentally different from those in breastmilk.

Breastmilk boosts a newborn baby's immature immune system.

Because a mom and her breastfeeding baby are usually together, their bodies are exposed to the same germs. Mom's immune response to germs puts specific, helpful antibodies into her breastmilk. When she nurses, these antibodies help strengthen her baby's immune system.

Breastfeeding provides comfort.

Breastfeeding gives mom a handy tool for calming her baby when he's fussy, or for soothing him to sleep.

Breastfeeding promotes normal development of the face and jaw.

Bottlefeeding, on the other hand, increases the likelihood a child will experience dental problems or need speech therapy or orthodontia later. Bottlefeeding also increases the risk of snoring and the development of related breathing problems.

Breastfeeding promotes normal vision development.

The distance between the eyes of a baby at the breast and his mother's eyes is about 10 inches, exactly the distance for the sharpest focus and clearest vision for a young infant.

Breastfeeding may help to establish a healthy body weight.

Breastfed babies take only the amount of milk they need. This helps develop healthy eating patterns and may help prevent obesity. Studies have also found a connection between formula feeding and higher cholesterol levels in adulthood.

Breastfeeding promotes normal development in other areas on the health and wellness spectrum.

Studies have found connections between formula feeding and a *slightly* increased risk of ear infections, sinus infections, gastro-intestinal upsets, respiratory-tract infections, asthma, diabetes, Crohn's disease, celiac disease, ulcerative colitis, and other medical concerns.

Risk factors for these illnesses are multi-factorial, however, so breastfeeding is just one of many ways to bolster your baby's health.

Breastfeeding gives mom's health a boost.

Every month of breastfeeding makes a ***slight*** contribution to reducing a woman's lifetime risk of heart disease, diabetes, osteoporosis, and certain cancers (breast, ovarian, cervical, and uterine). Breastfeeding also helps your uterus return to normal size, and releases hormones that help you relax.

Breastfeeding, once established, is convenient for mom.

Bottlefeeding involves measuring, mixing, heating, sterilizing, cleanup, and dealing with leftovers—all of which is avoided with breastfeeding. Bottlefeeding also involves greater sleep deprivation since you have to be fully awake to prepare and serve a bottle at night.

For these reasons, many moms find that breastfeeding, once it is established (after baby is four to six weeks old), is easier and simpler than bottlefeeding. A baby can be breastfed anywhere, anytime. Your breastmilk is always fresh, it's always the right temperature, and you always have just the right amount available.

Breastfeeding seeds beneficial bacteria in baby's intestinal tract.

A newborn baby's intestine isn't fully developed at birth, so it needs the protection that breastmilk provides.

The bacteria introduced into our guts in infancy have a lasting impact on our health. One study found that nearly a third of the beneficial bacteria in a baby's intestinal tract come directly from mother's milk, and an additional 10 percent come from skin on the mother's breast.[48] Another study found that while the gut microbiome contin-

---

[48] Pia S. Pannaraj, Fan Li, Chiara Cerini, Jeffrey M. Bender, Shangxin Yang, Adrienne Rollie, Helty Adisetiyo, Sara Zabih, Pamela J. Lincez, Kyle Bittinger, Aubrey Bailey, Frederic D. Bushman, John W. Sleasman, Grace M. Aldrovandi. "Association Between Breast Milk Bacterial Communities and Establishment and Development of the Infant Gut Microbiome." *JAMA Pediatrics* (2017);

ues to experience variations throughout life due to diet, environment, lifestyle, genetics, and physiological state, the *first* micro-organisms to arrive in our gut after birth have the highest level of staying power and the strongest influence on how the gut microbiome develops.[49]

The intestinal tract's microbiome matters because poor gut health has been linked to obesity, Type 2 diabetes, heart disease, inflammatory bowel disease, colon cancer, neurological disorders, autism, allergies, and immune-system strength. A growing body of research is also finding a relationship between gut health and brain health; namely, between the absence of certain gut microbes and depression.

Because the first bacteria introduced in our guts have a lasting impact on our health, moms who breastfeed for even just the first few days after birth are able to provide their babies with a good dose of macrobiotics that can persist into adulthood.

Breastmilk is the baseline.

I purposefully framed the list above as "reasons breastfeeding is recommended by health professionals," rather than as a list of the "benefits of breastfeeding," because it would be misleading to say breastfeeding is "beneficial" to babies and moms. It isn't extra special or extra good: it's simply what we're wired to do. Human infants are biologically designed to thrive on breastmilk.

Laying the groundwork while you're pregnant.

Here are four concrete things you can do to prepare for breastfeeding before baby arrives.

---

[49] Inés Martínez, Maria X Maldonado-Gomez, João Carlos Gomes-Neto, Hatem Kittana, Hua Ding, Robert Schmaltz, Payal Joglekar, Roberto Jiménez Cardona, Nathan L Marsteller, Steven W Kembel, Andrew K Benson, Daniel A Peterson, Amanda E Ramer-Tait, Jens Walter, "Experimental evaluation of the importance of colonization history in early-life gut microbiota assembly." *eLife* 2018;7:e36521 DOI: 10.7554/eLife.3652 (2018)

First, talk to mothers who have met their breastfeeding goals.

Ask another momma to share her breastfeeding experiences and challenges with you. What were the biggest surprises, good and bad? What does she wish she'd known?

Secondly, sit with a mother while she breastfeeds.

If this seems awkward—watching another woman use her breast to feed a baby—you can compare it to riding a bicycle. If you'd only ever read about how to ride a bicycle and had never ever actually *seen* a person riding one, would you be able to figure it all out just from the written text? The balancing, the pedalling, the positioning of your legs, arms, and torso relative to one another? It'd be mighty difficult. Breastfeeding uses the same side of your brain as bicycle riding. You need to see it to get it.

If you don't personally know anyone who is currently breastfeeding, attend a local support group. To find one near you, ask your doctor, your midwife, or visit the La Leche League website. Pregnant moms are always welcome at La Leche League gatherings; it's not just for mommas whose babies have already arrived.

Another option: watch the videos on Dr. Jack Newman's website at ibconline.ca/breastfeeding-videos-english/ (the International Breastfeeding Centre).

Thirdly, talk to your partner about breastfeeding.

Have a candid discussion about your breastfeeding goals. Is your goal to breastfeed for a few days? A few weeks? Or are you hoping to breastfeed exclusively for the first half year? Does your partner know that breastfeeding is something you plan to do?

Sometimes new dads suggest throwing in the towel when things aren't coming easy in the first few days. Encourage your partner to become familiar with the breastfeeding process. If you share the same goals and information, then your partner can be a great source of strength and protection.

And finally, have an emergency support person lined up.

If the going gets rough, it can help to have someone to talk to—someone who understands breastfeeding and who hasn't just had a baby. This means someone other than dad. He's just had a baby, too, and he's just as frazzled as you are.

Getting started: Breastfeeding your newborn baby

Here are the three breastfeeding basics for a newborn baby.

One: Skin-to-skin.

"Skin-to-skin" contact means holding baby tummy to mommy with him wearing only a diaper, and you topless. During the first 4-6 weeks after birth, spend as many hours as possible skin-to-skin. Some people call this intense time together a "babymoon."

Two: Reclined.

Lean back to nurse, the way you recline in bed to read a book or when you're flaked out on the couch in front of the TV. When your newborn breastfeeds tummy-on-mommy, gravity will help bring him in for a nice, deep latch. Newborns nurse longer when they have a deep latch, and moms are less likely to experience nipple damage. Yay, gravity![50]

Three: Early and often.

Try to latch baby around an hour after birth, then continue to nurse as often as possible.

---

[50] To get a sense of what laidback nursing looks like, have a look at Dr. Suzanne Colson's website, or check out this excerpt from the classic book *The Womanly Art of Breastfeeding*: lllc.ca//sites/default/files/Laid-back-bf_WAB.pdf.

The science: How often is "often"?

It doesn't always make sense to use numbers when it comes to frequency of nursing a newborn baby.

Perhaps a little biology lesson might help to explain just how much a newborn baby needs to feed. In 2013, I attended a presentation by eminent breastfeeding expert Nancy Mohrbacher at an LLLC Health Professional Seminar in Calgary.[51] Her presentation included a visual breakdown of how patterns of nursing frequency in newborn mammals are determined by maturity at birth and composition of milk. Learning about nursing frequency differences in cache mammals (e.g., deer, seals, rabbits) versus carry mammals (e.g., apes, marsupials) helped me understand why newborn human babies nurse so often.

Mohrbacher pointed out that cache mammals feed about every 12 hours on milk that is quite high in protein and fat. The offspring of dears, seals and rabbits, for example, spend long hours tucked away in hiding spots, away from their grazing and feeding mommas.

Follow mammals (e.g., giraffes, cows) feed more often than cache mammals and have milk lower in fat and protein.

Nest mammals (e.g., dogs, cats) feed every couple of hours and have milk that is even lower in fat and protein.

Carry mammals (e.g., apes, marsupials) feed around the clock. Their milk is lower still in fat and protein.

Of all mammalian milks, human milk is among the lowest in fat and protein.

No wonder human newborns have a biological need to nurse so frequently!

---

51 You'll find excellent breastfeeding resources, including information on how to download Nancy Mohrbacher's Breastfeeding Solutions app, at: nancymohrbacher.com.

The math: How often is "often"?

You might be thinking, *I sort of get it, but come on, give me a number. I need a yardstick. How often is "often"?*

A long time ago, moms were told to nurse a newborn baby for 20 minutes on each side, but we now know that trying to time nursings can make it harder for a mom to reach her breastfeeding goals. After all, with a newborn baby you never know whether any individual nursing session will last four minutes or four hours (or any length of time in between).

Then, a few years back, experts started telling moms to nurse every two hours. But that's not helpful either, because, again, every time a nursing session ends with a newborn, you never know if the next one will begin in five minutes or in five hours (or any length of time in between).[52]

More recently, many moms have been told to expect to nurse their baby eight to 12 times per day. Again, though, this number makes it harder for some moms to get comfortable with breastfeeding, because with a breastfeeding newborn it can be hard to differentiate between discrete nursing sessions. For example, if a baby falls asleep while nursing on one side, and stays latched on, and then wakes up an hour later and starts suckling actively on that same breast again—does this count as one breastfeeding session or two?

So, really, numbers can do more harm than good when you're breastfeeding a newborn. But if you *must* have a number—if that number will help reassure you that you're doing it right—then how about this: you can expect that, in the first few days after birth, breastfeeding will consume around eight hours out of each 24-hour period.

That's right. Eight hours out of 24 during the first few days.

---

[52] Sometimes doctors advise moms to breastfeed a medically vulnerable baby every two hours at a minimum. If this applies to your case, ask your health professionals when you can stop scheduling the feedings this way. Some moms mistakenly continue to wake their babies every two hours for a feeding long after there's a medical need for it, simply because they were never given permission to stop.

Breastfeeding eight hours per day: Holy moly!

Let's be realistic—having a little person latched on your breast for eight out of every 24 hours brings with it some challenges and sacrifices: physical discomfort, fractured sleep, and unbalanced caregiving between you and your partner.

Just try to keep in mind that this is not permanent. Soon enough, your baby will become more efficient at nursing and your milk supply will increase to its maximum capacity. As your baby and your body hit these milestones, the amount of time you spend each day on breastfeeding will decrease substantially.

In the meantime, though, getting comfortable with breastfeeding a newborn means nursing *a lot*. It's a commitment. Remember, your baby was used to being fed continuously while in the womb. It takes time to transition from continuous feeding to the adult standard of three discrete mealtimes per day.

> "The sun, with all those planets revolving around it and dependent upon it, can still ripen a bunch of grapes as if it had nothing else in the universe to do."
>
> — Galileo Galilei, physicist and astronomer (1564-1642)

When I hear moms wistfully explain that they couldn't breastfeed because they just didn't make enough milk, or that their milk supply just "dried up" on its own a couple of months in, I suspect that, for the most part, it's because no one ever told them that they should expect to breastfeed for about eight out of every 24 hours to get things started. The vast majority of women are physically capable of making enough breastmilk for their babies—they just need someone to give them accurate information about what it takes to make that happen.

Breastfeeding is natural, we're told. Well, yes, it is.

The corollary, of course, is that it's damn hard to get it going.

You may be having second thoughts about breastfeeding right about now.

Maybe Plan A was for you and your spouse to alternate night feedings and divvy up this parenting gig equally.

I'm not saying you can't do that. This is your family. You get to make the call. You shouldn't be forced into breastfeeding by some unbending constraint of biological determinism.

I'm just saying that if you choose to share feeding duties with other family members in the first few weeks, then you're unlikely to reach your breastfeeding goals.

You and your spouse may be devoted to gender equality, but newborn babies aren't. Given this immutable reality, you have to decide whether it works for your family to temporarily quell your egalitarian principles for the sake of breastfeeding.

So, reflect on this a bit: How do *you* feel about the prospect of nursing for around eight hours per day for the first few days and close to that amount for the first few weeks after birth?

Some moms willingly embrace the full-on commitment required to breastfeed a baby. They see it as a temporary extension of the one-sided effort that nature foists upon mothers in growing and birthing a baby.

Other moms find the one-sidedness of breastfeeding—from mom, just mom, always mom, never from the other parent—too much of a submission, a surrender, a sacrifice, a capitulation.

Realistically, breastfeeding a baby *is* a form of submission, surrender, sacrifice, capitulation. It just is. You lose. Dad wins. Unfair.

But resisting this submission can sometimes make the newborn phase harder. Pregnancy and early motherhood disrupt your life in a way that's hard to gloss over.

Even without near-constant breastfeeding, there's a new, highly unproductive, stop-and-start rhythm to get used to. Baby wants this, baby needs that. Baby needs a diaper. Baby needs to sleep. Baby needs to eat. Pick baby up. Put baby down. Children always need something from you. It's why American comedian and late-night talk show host Stephen Colbert adroitly describes them as "small but relentless opponents." Relentless, indeed.

These intermittent but constant interruptions can take us out of a focused, productive work state and induce overwhelming lethargy: you just can't get anything done. *Ugh.*

If you're not willing to adapt to this reality and keep your expectations low, early motherhood can turn into an anxiety-inducing, joyless, and dreary experience.

But if you can give in for a short while, you might better enjoy the sweetness of the new-baby phase, which somehow, simultaneously, feels both liminal and brief.

The all-in newborn phase, the intense growing-baby phase, the need-to-be-always-vigilant toddler phase will soon all be over. The further you move from your child's birth day, the less you matter. With every passing day, there's more and more that dads and grandparents and babysitters can do to pitch in. It seems hard to believe now, but your other identities *will* come back. You'll return to the other side. You'll feel like yourself again. Not just somebody's mother—but *you*.

Breastfeeding a baby doesn't mean the division of household labour will be unequal forever. It certainly doesn't mean that you need to become a baby-centred, one-dimensional mama bear from now on. But it's easier to make breastfeeding work if you have a clear-eyed, realistic understanding that it involves the willingness—temporarily—to go all in.

And it's not like you need to give up on the ideal of parental equality if you choose to breastfeed.

Get your partner[53] to change diapers! And give baths! And stick baby in the baby carrier and go for a walk during the evening fussies!

A few more good ones: In about a year, you can get your partner to pitch in equally with daycare drop-offs/pickups/leaving-an-important-meeting-to-grab-baby-at-10-am-when-the-daycare-

---

53   If you have one. Many parents have and raise babies solo these days.

calls-to-say-he-has-a-rash (a rash that the doctor subsequently informs you is inconsequential). Get dad to be responsible for remembering when swimming registration opens up. Get dad to figure out who the best local piano teacher is. Better yet, make it *dad's* job to oversee the piano *practice*, every day, forever. If there's an email list to sign up for or a form to fill out for a kid activity, make your partner the default parent to get that email and fill out that form. Nail trimming! New-winter-boot shopping! Playdate organizing!

If you want to set up a dynamic where both your careers are of equal importance, be aware that any schmo will step up in the first few weeks when the baby is new and exciting. For most families, true gender equality breaks down way past the milk-feeding stage.

Ages and Stages

So let's say, after reading all that, you decide you're still in: Your plan is to breastfeed. Here's a recap of how breastfeeding evolves as your baby moves past the newborn stage.

First 40 days

After you've diligently established breastfeeding by following the Breastfeeding Basics,[54] breastfeeding continues to be "on demand" both day and night for the first six weeks.

Six weeks to six months

Around the age of six weeks, babies become far more efficient at nursing and figure out, on their own, how to feed less often and for shorter sessions while still taking in the same volume of milk.

Your body becomes more efficient at producing breastmilk, too. Your breasts feel less full, you stop leaking milk, you no longer feel the

---

[54] Breastfeeding Basics: (1) skin-to-skin; (2) reclined position; (3) early and often; and, apparently, (4) *temporarily* ditching your deep-seated faith in gender equality.

milk ejection, and the milk looks thin and almost blue. None of this means your milk is "drying up." It's all just part of the normal course of breastfeeding.

Another change: While breastfeeding continues to be "on demand" throughout the daytime, at night it's now a different story. You now have the earliest opportunity to partially night-wean your healthy, full-term baby to sleep through a four-to-six-hour stretch at night (see Chapter 7).

Six months

The daytime weaning process begins at around five or six months of age, when your baby starts solids. At this stage, there's nothing you need to change or do differently to begin the weaning process. With every bite of solid food your baby takes in, your body gets the message and makes less milk.

Nine months

At nine months of age, if they wish, parents can fully night-wean their baby, which means no nursing between bedtime and the morning wake-up.

12 months

While full-term nursing goes to at least 15 months of age, once they hit 12 months, babies no longer need to be nursed "on demand" at any time, day or night. At this point, mommas have 100 percent control in terms of setting the rules around where, when, and for how long they choose to nurse.

15 months

Full-term nursing continues to a minimum of 15 months, during which breastmilk—or a breastmilk substitute such as formula—is a biological necessity. Replacing breastmilk or formula with plain cow's milk before 15 months can lead to nutritional deficiencies in your baby.

Just to be clear—it's perfectly fine to include cow's milk in your baby's diet once solids are introduced at the age of six months, but the milk should be offered in a cup (*not a bottle or sippy cup*) or as an ingredient in a dish you are serving. Cow's milk on its own is not a replacement for breastmilk or formula.

2 years and beyond

Breastfeeding—complemented by solid foods on a plate and beverages in a cup—can continue up to two years of age or beyond.

The normal course of weaning

The easiest way to fully wean a child off breastmilk is to do it so subtly that he's not even aware he's being weaned.

Chapters 12, 13, and 14 have information to help make the full weaning process go as smoothly as possible. The breastfeeding websites and other resources listed at the end of this book also offer information on weaning.

Breastmilk in a bottle

At some point, pretty well every momma[55] needs to take some time away from baby, whether because of a need to work, a dental appointment, or an evening out with friends. Whatever the reason, absences are inevitable. This section has some tips for getting time away from baby and giving him expressed breastmilk in a bottle.

Shelf life of breastmilk

Human milk, like all foods, loses some of its nutritional qualities when refrigerated—and more when it's frozen. For that reason, freshly

---

[55] I say "momma," because I assume daddy has already figured out how to take time away from baby, without even reading this book. Clever, clever daddies. How *do* they do it?

pumped room-temperature breastmilk has more nutritional value than refrigerated or frozen breastmilk.

> **Good to know!**
>
> Expressed breastmilk can safely last four to six hours at room temperature, three to eight days in the refrigerator, and two to 12 months in a home freezer.

A mother's expressed breastmilk can be safely stored at room temperature for four to six hours, though some studies suggest it can be safely stored on the kitchen counter for as long as ten hours! Freshly expressed human milk can be stored at room temperature longer than the cow's milk you buy at the store because it's a fresh, living substance that contains antibodies and live cells that discourage the growth of bad bacteria.

In other words, as long as you're not in the middle of a summer heat wave, you can feel confident about expressing shortly before you head out, and then leaving your breastmilk in a sealed container on the kitchen counter, ready to go. Babies are fine with room-temperature milk, which means your baby's caregiver won't even need to heat the bottle before serving it.

Practice makes perfect? Naaah….

Contrary to popular myth, there's no need to "practise" giving baby a regular bottle so he gets used to it.

If you offer your baby a bottle once per week or less there's still a chance he'll reject it at some point anyway, in which case all that forced weekly pumping and bottle-feeding will be for naught.

If, on the other hand, you offer a bottle more than once per week, you not only risk your breastmilk supply dropping below what your baby needs, you also risk your baby rejecting your breast entirely for the easier-to-drink-from bottle.

Too few bottles: no good.

Too many bottles: no good.

What a bother!

Instead of arbitrarily scheduling practice times with a bottle, just keep things easy and only offer expressed human milk when the situation calls for it. You've got enough on your plate without sitting around while a wheezing, suctioned flange pulls at your nipple, just for the "practice."

And your Precious Little Petunia Bottom does not need practice with a regular bottle. You've given birth to an indubitable genius! No practice needed here. Your baby's too smart to starve just because momma has stepped out for the evening.

Tips for serving expressed breastmilk

Many breastfed babies throw a fit if momma tries to bottle-feed. The good news is that this means mom is off the hook for bottle-feeding. It's not your problem. Your baby's caregiver is perfectly capable of figuring it out. Have faith in dad or the nanny.

Some tips to set up dad or the babysitter for success:

- ✓ **Nurse baby right before you step out the door.** A fed baby is a happy baby.

- ✓ **Ask your baby's caregiver to offer the first expressed-milk feeding soon after you leaves.** A recently fed baby is a baby who is more amenable to trying something weird and new. If your caregiver waits until baby is hangry, then their chances of success decrease exponentially. Remember, babies LOVE to put stuff in their mouth—so why not a bottle nipple, right!?

- ✓ **Your caregiver has other options.** If your baby isn't keen on expressed milk in a bottle, then your caregiver has other options: a spoon, an open cup, a feeding syringe, or a dropper.

- ✓ **Check guidelines for safely storing, thawing, and warming human milk, and dealing with leftovers.** On the La Leche League Canada website, you'll find detailed information about storing and serving expressed human milk, which you can provide to your caregiver.

One more tip if you're heading out the door and leaving a bottle behind for your partner:

Dads.
Never.
Babysit.

They parent.

Partial breastfeeding/partial bottle-feeding

It can be hard to strike a balance between a bit of breastfeeding and a bit of bottlefeeding.

Breastmilk supply is built up and then kept up on the basis of demand-and-supply. The less your baby nurses, the less milk your body produces. The less milk you make, the more frustrated your baby will be at the breast. Before long, he'll reject your unreliable breast entirely for the dependable, easier-to-use bottle.

For this reason, many moms find it simpler to go with one or the other—either full breastfeeding (with only the occasional bottle) or full formula (with perhaps a bit of that golden colostrum in the first few days).

Pumping and bottlefeeding isn't for everyone.

While parents often assume that breast pumps and bottles are indispensable with a baby in the house, you don't necessarily have to buy either of these items. Many families get through the baby stage just fine without ever using a breast pump or a bottle.

For example, if you limit your absences to two hours or fewer when baby is under six months, you won't need to leave a bottle behind when you head out the door. Breastfed newborns often prefer to wait for momma to return, rather than taking a bottle. Just nurse right before you leave, and then nurse again as soon as you get back. There are many ways your partner or another caregiver can entertain a newborn for a couple of hours while you're out. Carry baby. Smile at baby. Talk to baby. Go for a walk. Visit the grocery store. Visit the park. Food isn't the only way to show love.

After the first six months, baby can have solid foods and water in a cup when you step out. Predictable daytime naps also make it easier to get out of the house without getting a bottle ready. And with baby's night bedtime starting as early as 6:30 pm by the time he's hit the half-year mark, there's now also plenty of time to squeeze in a late-night pub outing with friends or a date with your partner without the bother of leaving behind a bottle.

No pumping. No bottle washing. No drying pump parts cluttering up your kitchen counter. No dumping unused milk. No worries about messing with your milk supply.

Just one less thing to do.

Pump it up!

As with so many other aspects of parenting, though, it's different strokes for different folks. If you don't mind pumping, then you go, girl. Pump, pump it up!

Integrate your old life with your new life.

While some outings call for leaving your baby with daddy or grandparents or a babysitter, you can also start looking for opportunities to integrate various aspects of your life.

For example, there's no rule that says that you need to ship your kids out so you can have drinks with a friend. Sometimes, of course, it's more fun that way, but now that you have a baby you can also weave in some socializing that includes the kids.

> **Pro tip:**
>
> When a wedding or house-party invitation says "adults only," what they mean is that they don't want snot-nosed ingrates running around, screaming wildly, and smearing ketchup all over pristine walls. In other words, the prohibition applies to walking, talking children, and not babes in arms. Ask the hosts if you can bring your snoozy infant along—and assure them that you've hired a babysitter for your older kids.

If you look for natural opportunities to live your life without segregating family time and friend time, you might find the transition to parenthood a little smoother.

Drinking while breastfeeding

I only bring this up because the desire to have some guilt-free drinks with friends is sometimes the reason women start weaning early. The problem is, of course, that there's no ethical way to determine what amount of alcohol is safe for a breastfeeding mother to drink.

What we know is this:

a. It takes about 30 to 60 minutes for your liver to metabolize one standard alcoholic beverage and for alcohol to enter breastmilk.

b. It takes about two hours for the amount of alcohol in one standard drink to be eliminated from the body and leave breastmilk.

c. The more drinks you have, the higher your blood-alcohol concentration.

d. Breastmilk-alcohol concentration rises (and drops) at approximately the same rate as blood-alcohol concentration. In other words, when your blood-alcohol concentration is 0.08%, your breastmilk-alcohol concentration is at about 0.08%, too.

Obviously, since breastmilk-alcohol concentration rises and drops in the same way as blood-alcohol concentration, there's no need to pump and dump. You wouldn't try bloodletting to sober up, right? All you need is *time* to get the alcohol to break down and leave your system, which is why mothers are advised by some experts to wait two to three hours per drink before nursing—or better yet, to abstain entirely.[56]

That's what the experts say, anyway. The moms at my workshops who still go out on date nights say this: Because the alcohol level in your breastmilk is a small fraction of the alcohol level in the drinks you ingest, if you have one or two alcoholic beverages over the course of an evening, your baby might be getting the equivalent amount of

---

56 **See:** Canadian Centre on Substance Use and Addiction (CCSUA), *Canada's Guidance on Alcohol and Health: Final Report* (January 2023) ccsa.ca/canadas-guidance-alcohol-and-health

alcohol found in a few teaspoons of light beer (depending, of course, on various factors, such as your weight, baby's weight, the alcohol content in the beverages you're drinking, and how much breastmilk baby actually ends up ingesting in a nursing session). In other words, if your breastmilk-alcohol concentration is at about 0.08%, then it's like a 0.08% beer—a fraction of a 4.50% beer.

On top of that, your baby will consume the breastmilk orally and metabolize the alcohol before it hits his own bloodstream. (Although, just so you know, babies don't metabolize alcohol nearly as well as adults do.)

This is entirely different from drinking while pregnant. Alcohol goes straight from an expectant mom's bloodstream through her placenta. A fetus will therefore have the *same* blood-alcohol concentration as mom, which is why drinking alcohol during pregnancy is ill-advised. Having the occasional glass of wine before nursing isn't the same thing as drinking while pregnant.

Bottom line: alcohol use comes with risks for all people, nursing or not, and whether or not you imbibe is up to you.

If you want to partake of the odd drink while breastfeeding, here are some tips:

- ✓ Avoid alcohol entirely in the first 40 days after birth, when you're doing your most intense breastfeeding and baby is at his smallest weight. (The claim that Guinness will help bring in your milk is just an old wives' tale.)
- ✓ Consider low-alcohol beverages. Many craft breweries now make beers with alcohol content of 3.5% or less.
- ✓ Decide in advance how much you want to drink. If you're going to *stick to* a plan, you need to *come in with* a plan.
- ✓ To help keep track of your consumption, don't let servers or friends refill a half-empty glass.
- ✓ Drink a full pint of water between each alcoholic beverage to slow your pace.

✓ Eating helps to slow the passage of alcohol through your stomach, and aids in breaking it down before it reaches the liver. (It also gives your mouth something to do besides sipping.)

Persistent research results suggest that abstinence can cause greater health harm than moderate alcohol consumption. For those without alcohol abuse disorders—so, most of us—moderate alcohol consumption is a way to celebrate, relax, blow off steam with friends, and embrace the undulating joy of life. *L'chaim*! To life!

Speaking of food...

You can eat anything you want while breastfeeding. This includes spicy food, peanut butter, gluten, dairy, and coffee. Contrary to popular opinion, if your baby is fussy, gassy, rashy, or upset it's unlikely to be related to what you've been eating. As a result, restricting your diet is unlikely to fix anything.

Food gives us pleasure. Nursing mommas are allowed to have fun and eat strong flavours and spicy food. And your favourite foods will raise your spirits if you're dealing with a rashy, gassy, caterwauling baby.

The last word on breastfeeding

Breastfeeding is way more difficult than you ever imagined.

It's also much easier than you think.

Breastfeeding is very good for your baby. At the same time, it's also unnecessary, because babies do just fine with breastmilk substitutes.

Breastfeeding is yet another area of parenting where diametrically opposed concepts are simultaneously true. The best way to muddle through all the complexity is to figure out what works for you and leave the rest behind.

CHAPTER 17:

Sleep

> "Getting up too early is a vice habitual in horned owls, roosters, young children and freight trains. Some mommas acquire it from young children and some coffee pots from mommas."
>
> A paraphrasing inspired by Aldo Leopold's classic 1949 work *A Sand County Almanac*

This chapter provides an overview of sleep. It repeats some of the same information you'll find in the chronological, age-based chapters, but pulls together all the sleep-related bits so you can see the big picture of your sleep journey. Think of this as your sleep cheat sheet: all the basics, all in one spot.

In their first four months, babies sleep anytime, anywhere.

You cannot sleep-train a baby less than 12 to 16 weeks old to follow a set bedtime schedule. Throughout the first three or four months you'll have no idea, once baby falls asleep, how long he'll stay asleep. You'll also have no idea, once baby wakes up, when his next nap will be.

> **Good to know!**
>
> To prevent choking and smothering, keep toys and pillows out of the bassinet or crib.

Nurse your newborn to sleep whenever you observe signs of sleepiness (eye rubbing, yawning, crankiness after a diaper change or feeding), which you can usually—but not always—expect after one to two hours of wakefulness.

Consider acquiring a bassinet.

At night, most parents find it practical to have their newborn sleep next to them in a bassinet in their bedroom.

Learn the best practices for sharing a sleep surface, even if you plan to never co-sleep.

Almost every mother will accidentally fall asleep with her baby in her arms at some point, so you might as well have a safer sleep surface set up for when that happens. Chapter 18 outlines the basics for co-sleeping.

<u>Do</u> let your newborn baby sleep in your arms.

In many cultures around the world, moms and babies share a "babymoon" together for the first 40 days or so after birth. A babymoon involves mom relaxing, reclined, with baby on her chest, bare-skin-to-bare-skin. Because newborn babies sleep 16 to 17 hours per 24-hour day, once they're cuddled against momma, there's a high probability they'll spend most of their time slumbering.

<u>Don't</u> let your baby sleep in your arms—at least not when *you're* sleeping.

Having baby sleep directly on your chest is lovely—as long as you're awake. But *you* need at least six to seven hours of sleep each night, which is hard to do with a hot, snuffling, snorting baby directly on top of you.

And if you're wondering why co-sleeping is okay, but spending all night with baby sleeping on top of you is *not*, keep in mind that sleeping on your chest isn't the same as sharing a sleep surface. When families choose co-sleeping, mom and baby tend to spend most of the night curled up *next* to each other, not *on top* of one another.

If you feel breastfeeding is going well and health professionals are happy with your baby's growth, then <u>after about two weeks</u> you can gently ease into being less responsive at night.

You cannot train a baby under the age of 40 days to sleep through the night. You *can*, however, gently nudge baby towards self-weaning at night by being ***slower to respond***. You still need to respond, mind you, just not as promptly.

It's a fine art. You cannot leave a baby between the ages of 14 days and 40 days to cry and cry, but neither do you have to jump up to nurse baby back to sleep the moment you hear him sniffle. Take a minute. Or two. Or ten, if you're exhausted.

If you feel breastfeeding is going well and health professionals are happy with your baby's growth, then you can try partially night-weaning baby any time <u>after 40 days</u>, if you want to.

Night-weaning means getting your baby accustomed to not being fed throughout the night. You'll find detailed instructions on this process in Chapter 7. Keep in mind that it takes several nights, that it *does* require effort from both mom and dad, and that it *will* involve crying. Because tears are involved, parents should only embark on this journey if they're truly committed to reclaiming a four- to six-hour period of uninterrupted sleep at night.

When he's around two months, baby will move up his night bedtime.

If your newborn was falling asleep between 10 pm and midnight, sometime around two months he will naturally begin to develop an earlier bedtime, likely between 9 and 11 pm. And then around three months he'll likely, on his own, move bedtime to between about 8 and 10 pm. This is a baby-led (not parent-led) phenomenon.

SLEEP

When baby is between three and four months, ease off on the mobile naps.

After four months of age, car rides, strollers, swings, baby carriers, or your arms should be the exception—not the rule—for getting your baby to sleep. Past the newborn stage, it's hard for a baby to have a deep, restful sleep on the go.

When baby is around three to five months, you can establish set bedtimes.

Around this age, baby is ready to consolidate his many daytime sleeps into two or three daytime naps at predictable times. Getting your baby used to a routine bedtime schedule is called ***sleep-training***. The process of setting up a sleep schedule *does* involve effort by mom and dad, and it often involves crying, but the payoff is a baby who's well rested, easygoing, and happy.

Sleep-training and night-weaning have nothing to do with disciplining a child.

Look at it this way: the same families who night-wean and sleep-train would never leave their child to "cry it out" as punishment for something they did while fully awake. Night-weaning and sleep-training have nothing to do with discipline. They're just about sleep.

Sleep-training and night-weaning do no harm.

Some critics warn that partially night-weaning between six and 12 weeks and then sleep-training between three and five months will instill a sense of abandonment, discourage communication, and teach a baby that his parents are irredeemable, unresponsive felons.

That's utter nonsense.

Not a single study has ever come even close to making this case.

Millions of night-weaned and sleep-trained babies gurgling joyfully at wake-up time demonstrate that age-appropriate night-weaning and sleep-training do no harm.

A rested baby is a happy baby.

A rested momma is a happy momma, too.

Yaaaasss queen, yas! Momma. Is. Going. To. Get. Some. Sleep. Yas!

Seriously, no harm done.

When sleep-training critics cite studies claiming that leaving babies to cry results in emotional, behavioural, or physical harm, they're referencing studies that examined a *chronic* pattern of caregiver non-responsiveness to crying. In other words, they're talking about studies of vulnerable children, including abandoned children raised in orphanages, or neglected children who've been removed from the custody of their parents. Studies of children who have experienced trauma and negligent caregiving amply demonstrate that children who are regularly left to cry will experience toxic stress levels, which in turn increases their risk for developing social-attachment disorders, behavioural issues, and abnormal stress reactions later in life.

It is frankly irresponsible that fearmongers extrapolate data from extreme, sad cases to conclude that any amount of crying, ever, must be strictly avoided. Four or five nights of nighttime crying until he drifts off to sleep is nowhere near the same thing as ignoring a fully awake baby in a crib for hours on end, every single day, for months at a time. There is a difference between toxic stress and tolerable stress.

Well, can you *prove* to me that sleep-training isn't harmful?

Around a century ago, the idea somehow emerged that we need science to guide us through loving and caring for our babies. We started to think of breastfeeding and sleeping as some sort of primitive claptrap to overcome. What I am asking you to do is to go about babycare as your great-great-great-grandmother would have gone about it and see sleeping through the night not as the problem, but as the cure.

As the momma, *you* get to make the choices for your own family and you are allowed to care for your baby the way babies are meant to be cared for: without fear or guilt, and with delight.

So, instead of obsessively searching for lab-controlled, easily replicated scientific proof that sleep-training isn't harmful, I'm going to turn things around and say this: Show me the lab-controlled, easily replicated scientific proof that it *is* harmful. Can't find it? That's because there isn't any.

It's the no-cry sleep solution!

I want to let you in on something really important: Babies who are sleep-trained to have a regular bedtime schedule and who are night-weaned to sleep through the night almost *never* cry.

This is an important point to drive home. Sleep-training and night-weaning *reduce* crying; they don't *increase* crying!

Unfortunately, there is a misconception that sleep-training and night-weaning result in babies wailing and crying themselves to sleep *every* night, which is why these effective, time-honoured techniques have fallen out of favour among a certain (attachment-parenting) crowd.

I have a pretty good idea how this misconception came about: it's because books that cover sleep—this one included—focus on the tricky transitional periods, and not the regular day-to-day. Around the ages of 40 days, four months, nine months, and 20 months, sleep-training and night-weaning briefly involve crying, yes, but that's it.

Other than those brief training and weaning periods, babies who are sleep-trained and night-weaned fall asleep every nap and every night without a sniffle. It may seem counter-intuitive and ironic, but age-appropriate night-weaning and sleep-training are the true no-cry sleep solutions!

Night-waking is normal and expected.

We all (adults, children, babies) wake up several times each and every single night as part of our natural sleep cycles. *After successful sleep-training*, it's to be expected that your baby will continue to occasionally wake up and then be unable to fall back asleep on his own because he needs mom or dad to look after his needs (relief from the stuffiness of a cold, soothing after a nightmare, dealing with the excitement of a recent trip, or hitting a major developmental milestone). Feel free to nurse your baby at night when this happens. Comforting him builds trust.

Night-weaning doesn't mean you'll never nurse at night again. It just means that night-nursing will become a sweet, special, exceptional event.

Past the infant stage, keep the bedtime routine brief.

Once you have sleep-trained baby to follow a scheduled morning nap, scheduled afternoon nap, and scheduled evening bedtime, keep the soothing-to-sleep routine as brief as possible. If the soothing-to-sleep routine you've chosen is taking an hour (regardless of what it involves—breastfeeding, singing lullabies, rubbing baby's back, rocking, or anything, really), then it's no longer working for you. And hey, if your soothing-to-sleep routine is taking that long, then it's no longer working for your baby, either. You need to keep things moving, Momma.

Allow yourself exceptions.

Many moms feel trapped by the nap. The good news: Once it's well established, you can make exceptions and skip the occasional nap here and there. Your child will be cranky when he misses a nap, but sometimes it's worth it for the greater good of a family adventure.

Around 12 months of age, babies drop their morning nap.

Dropping the morning nap is somewhat disruptive. Baby will be cranky for a few months because he'll be in a stage where "two naps are too many and one isn't enough." Plus, there's suddenly a major chunk of the day where baby is awake.

Mobile and awake.

Mobile, awake, destructive, accident-prone, and cranky.

Fun, fun!

Babies drop their morning nap on their own—there's nothing mom or dad needs to do to make this process happen. You can find more information on this process in Chapter 12.

Around 20 to 24 months, toddlers stage a "nap strike."

This is a normal developmental milestone, because your child is gaining awareness that *everything fun* happens while he's sleeping. It's just a classic case of FOMO.

Chapter 13 has suggestions for helping junior get back on track—his body still needs those naps.

An early afternoon nap never interferes with a good night's sleep.

A well-rested child has an easier time falling asleep. Lack of sleep leads to a child feeling overtired and wired.

If your toddler suddenly has trouble falling asleep at night, it's not because of his afternoon nap (unless that afternoon nap is happening too late in the day). Some potential solutions:

- ✓ Double check that the afternoon nap is starting early enough—aim to start the soothing routine at noon.
- ✓ Perhaps the bedroom needs darker curtains to block light.
- ✓ Even though it sounds counter-intuitive, try moving baby's night bedtime earlier—as early as 6:30 pm.
- ✓ Do nothing. Even the best sleeper will sometimes protest bedtime for a week or two for some random reason.

Don't rush to get out of the crib.

Aim to keep your toddler in the crib until well past 24 months. If he's not yet trying to climb *out* of the crib, just keep using it. (Toddlers figure out how to climb *into* the crib a lot sooner than they learn how to climb out.)

There are three main reasons to hang onto the crib:

1. *It's the safest place for your toddler.* Occasionally you hear reports of tragic accidents that happen in the middle of the night, but which parents don't discover until morning. A toddler who left and then was locked out of an apartment building in the middle of winter, or a two-year-old who drowned in a toilet.

A crib provides a safe space that helps contain your curious, growing baby.

2. *Your toddler finds it cozy.* The crib is like a familiar little nest that's just the right size for baby. If you always pick up your child promptly (or fairly promptly) after he wakes, then there'll be no reason for him to either: (a) feel negative about being in the crib; or (b) attempt to climb out of it.

3. *You'll save money.* Skip the whole "toddler bed" purchase and buy a real "big boy" bed that will get your child all the way through to when he grows up and moves out of your house one day (with said bed in tow).

Sometime after about 30 months (close to three years old), preschoolers begin slowly dropping their afternoon nap.

Dropping the afternoon nap is something that kids do on their own. There's nothing mom and dad need to do to make this process happen. Chapter 14 provides more detail about this development.

Once children drop their afternoon nap, they continue to fall asleep in the afternoon, *but on an intermittent basis*, until around the age of four or five.

Once your preschooler stops falling asleep in the afternoon, continue the afternoon nap *routine* for as long as possible.

Draw the curtains, perhaps read a story, and then leave the room. But before you leave, tell your child that he doesn't need to sleep if his body doesn't want to. Leave his bedroom door open so he can leave whenever he wants to. Hopefully he'll stay in bed playing with his stuffies for a bit, or flipping through the pages of a picture book, but it's okay if he doesn't. Leave it up to him.

There are three reasons to continue the afternoon nap routine after your child stops regularly falling asleep at naptime.

Firstly, he'll occasionally still need that afternoon nap, and continuing the nap routine gives him an opportunity to fall asleep at a reasonable time of day—closer to noon rather than in late afternoon.

Secondly, even if he doesn't fall asleep, a few minutes of quiet time will take the edge off of being awake all day. It also helps with emotional regulation: a young child who doesn't get a bit of quiet time in lieu of a nap is more at risk of being overwhelmed by the stress of his day and erupting into a temper tantrum.

Third reason: Mom and dad probably need the break!

Sleep is good. Good-quality sleep is a godsend.

For babies and toddlers—and, really, for all of us at any age—getting adequate sleep is important for mood regulation and maintaining positive social interactions. It's among the most critical factors for memory consolidation, productivity, cognitive development, and immune function. It affects our food decisions and our ability to problem solve. Researchers are also beginning to find links between childhood sleep deprivation and insomnia, depression, and learning disorders such as ADHD.

The effects of sleep deprivation are relatively minor for some children, but they can be severe in others and we don't know who will be most susceptible. So why take the risk? Shielding our children's developing brains is one of our top priorities as parents. Sleep is essential to our health and survival.

CHAPTER 18:

The Ten Basics of Bed-Sharing

"Whatever gets you through the night."

Title of song written in 1974 by John Winston Lennon (1940 -1980)

Some families decide, right from the start, that bed-sharing isn't for them. 'S all right.

Some parents prefer to place their newborn baby in a bassinet and then move him to a crib around the middle of his first year. There are a number of reasons for making this choice. It's usually easier to night-wean when baby isn't sharing a sleep surface with you. Some parents find it uncomfortable to sleep with an extra body in the bed. There are also risks to bed-sharing, and some parents just don't want the stress of worrying about whether they've adequately mitigated those risks.

Other families decide, right from the start, to share a family bed. 'S all right.

Some moms choose bed-sharing because they find it easier to breast-feed at night, or simply because they like the closeness.

Regardless of whether you're planning to share a bed, it's good to at least review the basics of bed-sharing.

For one, even if it wasn't Plan A, you may end up deciding that bed-sharing is the best way to maximize your family's sleep. A few generations ago, people had much larger families in much smaller houses and the family bed was the norm. Experts estimate that at least a third of families end up with diverse sleeping arrangements, including in a family bed for all or part of the night.

Secondly, even if you're a committed non-bed-sharer, every breastfeeding mom will experience at least one occasion where she falls asleep while nursing her baby in the middle of the night. Your best bet is to create a spot for nighttime nursing that is set up to be as safe as possible in case you end up unintentionally falling asleep while breastfeeding.

Ten Bed-Sharing Basics

1. **Baby needs to be on his back.**
   Placing baby on his back is the safest position for him on every sleep surface.

2. **Baby needs to be healthy and full term**.
   If your baby is vulnerable, then you need to make a plan for how to avoid accidentally falling asleep while nursing at night.

3. **Baby needs to be appropriately dressed.**
   Babies who are too hot at night are at greater risk for a sudden unexpected death in infancy. This means no heavy duvets, either.

4. **Baby cannot be swaddled.**
   For safety reasons, a swaddled baby needs to sleep on his own separate sleep surface.

5. **Mom needs to exclusively breastfeed**.
   Moms who breastfeed naturally curl their bodies around their babies, with baby's head at breast level. The curled position, with mom on her side and her knees bent beneath baby, makes it almost impossible to roll over him.

Studies show, however, that moms who aren't breastfeeding *don't* tend to naturally stay in this safe position throughout the night. In other words, if you aren't exclusively breastfeeding, you're at greater risk of accidentally rolling over and suffocating your baby. If you sometimes nurse at the breast and sometimes bottle-feed, then you need to make a plan to avoid accidentally falling asleep while nursing at night.

Because dads and siblings aren't breastfeeding—and are therefore less sensitive to a newborn at night—mom should position herself between baby and anyone else who is sharing the bed.

6. **Everyone in the bed needs to be sober.**
   This prohibition includes drugs, as well.

7. **Make sure your bed is free of pets.**
   Bye, Fido and Mittens!

8. **Make sure your bed doesn't have a <u>soft surface</u> that poses a smothering risk.**
   You need to set up on a firm, flat surface, such as a mattress on the floor. No sofas or recliners, whose folds pose a smothering risk if baby rolls into them. No heavy blankets or loose bedding either. Make sure your baby cannot wriggle into or under a pillow. Tuck in any blankets around the firm mattress to avoid them shifting over and covering baby's head.

9. **Make sure your bed is free of <u>empty spaces</u> that pose a choking risk.**
   Check for any indentations or gaps where baby could get stuck. The danger isn't that baby will fall through head first, but that his small body will fall into an empty space and his larger head will get stuck, strangling him.
   A newborn's weak neck muscles mean there's also a risk of strangulation if his neck hangs over a gap.
   If you see any spaces between the bed's mattress and headboard or between the mattress and the sides of the bed, fill the cracks with tightly rolled-up towels or blankets.

10. **Consider distance to floor and landing surface.**

    To avoid long falls, consider setting up a mattress on the floor.

Some moms may find this a daunting list. Ten variables! Images of babies dangling and strangling!

Other moms may read it and think—oh yeah, I can totally do this. I can do *exactly* this.

Others will fall somewhere in the middle. They'll try to roughly address the ten variables just to be prepared—in a good enough sort of way—and resolve to avoid falling asleep with baby.

Different strokes for different folks.

Take some inspiration from bed-sharing families.

If bed-sharing isn't for you, at least consider taking some inspiration from bed-sharing families. Some questions to think about:

- ✓ What can you do to minimize the distance you have to travel around your house to nurse at night? The closer you can stay to your bed, the less you'll be roused during the nighttime feeding, and the easier it will be for you to fall back asleep.

- ✓ Instead of a nursing couch, can you nurse on a safely arranged spare bed at night, so that baby is safer if you accidentally fall asleep?

- ✓ If your partner (who presumably has to get to work in the morning) is disturbed by nighttime nursing, can one of you sleep somewhere else in the house on a temporary basis? At least until baby is night-weaned?

- ✓ Are you open to making different sleep arrangements for different parts of the night? For example, some moms aren't comfortable co-sleeping all night, but are fine with dozing off in bed with their little one with them after the super-early-morning feed that many babies want around 4 or 5 am.

CHAPTER 19:

The Twelve Most Frequently Asked Questions

To round out the Troubleshooting section of this book, here are the Top 12 questions that you'll be asked throughout your pregnancy and during your baby's first few years of life. Knowing these common questions ahead of time will help you prepare your answers.

Question #1: *"Have you set up the nursery yet?"*
Answer: *"Sure."*
The Low-Down:
There's actually not all that much you need to set up or buy before baby arrives.

People ask this question for two reasons.

First, it's their way of saying, "Oh, cool, you're expecting a baby! I'm excited for you and want to demonstrate my interest. This is my way of doing that."

The second reason is that they've bought into the standard marketing trope that loving parents would ensure, before baby arrives, that their home is well stocked with breast pumps, bottles, bottle warmers, a diaper bag, a nursing pillow, a hooter hider, a change table, bouncy chairs, educational toys, giraffe decals, bathtubs, diaper pails, sippy cups, a rocking chair, and baby-sized shoes. (Pro tip: every single item on the preceding list is something that you won't necessarily need during your baby's first year—or ever.)

Just answer a simple "yes" to this question, and then get into some other aspect of your life as an expectant momma. Share your ideas for names, or mention that your baby just started kicking… The person who asked about your nursery is simply giving you an opening to talk about what's new with your pregnancy and your preparations for the baby.

Question #2: *"Have you gotten away from the baby yet?"*
The Low-Down:
Before we had children, no one ever asked my husband and me whether we were regularly going out for date nights. (We weren't. We're homebodies.) Yet this has turned into a standard inquiry for new parents.

My best guess is that this question arose, in part, as a backlash to the attachment-parenting philosophy.

In case you're not familiar with it, attachment parenting basically takes a bunch of good ideas—breastfeeding, being responsive, using baby carriers—and subsumes them into an over-arching philosophy that also integrates a bunch of bad ideas—such as never, ever letting your baby cry. The implication is that if you follow the edicts of attachment parenting, you'll have a baby with a healthy attachment to his parents. If you fail to, you won't.

Of course, this is a bunch of hooey, and parents who don't take the attachment-parenting approach can't help but roll their eyes. After all, parents who don't breastfeed, don't own baby carriers, don't avoid sleep-training, don't co-sleep, and don't avoid upsetting their babies end up with children who are just as well attached.

It's also trying to watch attachment parents held captive by their young children. *Break free!*, many bystanders secretly yearn to tell them.

Yet it's hard to articulate opposition to attachment parenting. After all, if you're against attachment parenting, what are you *for*? Detached parenting? Aloof parenting? I-don't-give-a-damn parenting? How could anyone baldly state that they're not into attachment with their precious babies?

Journalist and fiction writer Leah McLaren brilliantly coined the term "semi-detached parenting" back in 2014, but somehow it never took off.[57] It should have.

Instead, asking if you'd "gotten away from your baby" has become a way of fishing out a new momma's parenting philosophy.

So, *have* you gotten away from your baby yet? Here are three possible answers:

Possible Answer #1: *"Oh no! I'd never dream of leaving my baby!"* gasps mom as she clutches her baby—the one she's already holding—even tighter. Okay, so now you know you're talking to an Attachment Parent.[58] Adjust your interactions accordingly.

Possible Answer #2: *"Oh yes! Next week my husband and I—just the two of us—are going to an all-inclusive resort!"* boasts mom, as she vigorously rocks the heavy car seat—the one with her wailing, four-week-old baby in it—back and forth and back and forth.
Okay, so not an Attachment Parent.

Possible Answer #3: *"Sure."*
Then give more details about how you're adjusting to life with baby. Take the question to mean: "So—you have a baby now! Pretty cool! Tell me more."

---

57   "Attachment parenting has been taken to the extreme. Here's my case for semi-detached," by Leah McLaren *The Globe and Mail:* May 22, 2014) This brief, brilliant, hilarious article is available at: theglobeandmail.com/life/parenting/a-guide-to-semi-detached-parenting/article18809304/

58   In defense of attachment parents everywhere, have a read of this very brief, brilliant, and hilarious article: "Confessions of an accidental attachment parent" by Susanna Schrobsdorff (*Time:* May 10, 2012). ideas.time.com/2012/05/10/confessions-of-an-accidental-attachment-parent/#ixzz1xM0OahtF.   Many attachment parents are lovely people.

Question #3: *"What's your baby's name?"*
Answer: *"Hester."*
The Low-Down:
I love the names Hester (for a girl) or Hoagy (for a boy), but my husband kiboshed these suggestions when we were expecting. I'm just putting them out there for you people.

In all seriousness, people will ask about your baby's name and gender not because we live in some sort of unbending patriarchy that's imposing a gender-normative order on everyone. Rather, people ask these two questions—boy or girl? name?—for one reason and one reason alone: Your baby is boring and *nooooo* other question comes to mind.

Don't get me wrong: Your baby is precious and probably the most beautiful baby every born. But he's also, so, so indistinguishable from every other baby. There's literally nothing else to ask about.

Except for, maybe….

Question #4: *"Is he a good baby?"*
Answer: *"Yes."*
The Low-Down:
When people ask this question, what they're trying to get at is: "Is your baby a quiet baby, or does your baby do an unbearable amount of crying?" A "good baby," so the thinking goes, would be one that never cried, and only nursed for 20 minutes every three hours, but never at night. In other words, a good baby would be one at risk for the dangerous classification known as "failure to thrive."

But, of course, the well-meaning person asking you this question isn't hoping you have a quiet newborn who's slowly starving to death.

Your best bet is to assume well-meaning intent with this question and provide a simple "yes." Begin with "yes," and then, only if you like, get into the details of how often he nurses at night, or whether he's treating you to a full-blown case of the evening fussies. Celebrate the fact that a "good baby" is one who makes his needs known loud and clear, so he can grow and meet developmental milestones.

When this question is asked, some moms like to turn to their babies and ask, "Whaddya say? Are you a good baby? *Are* you? Are you an actually pretty good baby? *Who'sagoodbaby?!*"

This will usually get a smile from your little one, which is, ultimately, all the asker was after. There's nothing like a bright baby smile to put the "good baby" question to rest.

Question #5: *"Is he a good sleeper?"*
Answer: *"Sure."*
The Low-Down:
"I'm using your answer to this question to determine whether you, Momma, have had enough sleep to make it worth my while to attempt a conversation with you," …is what some people might be thinking when they pose this tiresome query.

It implies that your baby's inherent nature determines whether he sleeps through the night or not, when, in reality, night-weaning past the age of about six weeks has more to do with mom and dad's tolerance for crying.

The alternative question is no good either: "Hey, Momma, are you a good sleep-trainer?" If mom says no, she'll be judged for being a wimp; if she says yes, she'll risk social opprobrium for her heartless cruelty. It's a lose-lose situation.

Bottom line: It's generally a good idea for people to keep their noses out of what goes on in your bedroom.

At best, *maybe*, it's okay for people to sympathetically ask you if you feel you're getting enough sleep.

(Spoiler alert: you aren't.)

Question #6: *"Is your baby teething?"*
Answer: *"You nailed it!"*
The Low-Down:
Any time your baby becomes slightly disgruntled or agitated, there's a possibility that some friendly soul will inquire after his dental status. For all you know, your baby is indeed teething, so you might as well say yes to the guess.

This question is usually intended as an invitation to gush more about your baby. Clearly this person is interested in the newest member of your family!

Question #7: *"Didn't you just nurse him?"*
Your Spoken-Out-Loud Answer: *"You're right, I totally did! It's soooo nice not be tied down to a schedule. I'm always ready for another cuddle with my little beanie."*
Your Inner-Voice Answer: "*Didn't you just have a beer/potato chip/ glass of wine/slice of cheesecake? And you're reaching for another one already?" (*eye roll*)*
The Low-Down:
This is more about the questioner's feelings and experiences than your parenting. Because the person you're speaking with doesn't have accurate information about what's involved in establishing and maintaining adequate milk supply, they assume breastfeeding is like a multi-vitamin—pop one and you'll be good for a while. Unless you're speaking with an expectant mother who genuinely wants you to explain nursing frequency so she can better understand this whole breastfeeding business, your best bet is to keep your response light and move on.

Question #8: *"How long are you going to breastfeed? Isn't he getting too old?"*
Answer: *"You're wondering when he's going to wean? I'm curious about that, too. I imagine he'll probably do it around the same age other kids wean off bottles. I'd love to know when he'll be done with soothers and diapers, too."*
The Low-Down:
Again, this question is more about the questioner's feelings and experiences than your parenting. The person you're speaking with is simply unfamiliar with the normal course of breastfeeding.

Questions about breastfeeding are supremely annoying. You're not breastfeeding to signal to the world that you're a sanctimonious mother who spends her days judging others for bottle-feeding. Honest to goodness, you're just breastfeeding your baby because you're breastfeeding your baby, and you want to be left alone. Being forced to defend or explain it can make you feel like you're nursing purely as a virtue-signalling exercise, when that's not the case at all.

Question #9: *"What do you do all day?"*
Your Spoken-Out-Loud Answer: *"Oh, you know, like with any job it's hard to explain the details to someone who isn't doing it."*
Your Inner-Voice Answer: *"If you're asking this question, then you just don't get it. You won't get it. Not even if I try to explain it to you. Let's just change the topic."*
The Low-Down:
Sometimes this question is asked by a woman expecting her first child because she's genuinely curious. Usually though, it comes from someone who has no experience being a stay-at-home parent and who pictures babycare as a monotonous vacation of daytime television broken up by frequent trips to the coffee shop with friends. It's best not to get into it. No one asks an engineer, a secretary, a retail worker, or plumber what she does all day, so there's no point in asking a momma on parental leave this question either.

Question #10: *"I read your book and none of it worked. I wasn't able to breastfeed, my baby isn't sleeping, and my toddler will only eat crackers. Can I have my money back?"*
Answer: *"Ha! Not going to happen."*
The Low-Down:
Oooh, sneaky. This is actually a question from a putative reader to me, and not a question a new mother would get, as I promised at the beginning of this section. But still, I'll answer it.

There are at least two reasons your baby experience wasn't "by the book."

First, you might actually have a unique baby on your hands. Why not? We can't all be the same. Uniformity is boring.

Secondly, consider this possibility: Operator error. Like, when it came time to sleep-train did you follow through with the crying, or was it too hard? There's no shame if you weren't able to let your baby cry until he fell asleep. But rather than saying, "I tried the cry-it-out method and it doesn't work," it may be more accurate to say, "I tried the cry-it-out method, but it doesn't work *for me*."

Question #11: *"What's for dinner?"*
Answer: *"Black bean gruel."*
The Low-Down:
Wait for it…wait for it….

Question #12: *"Mom, what's for dinner?"*
Answer: *"Ack! I just told you two minutes ago! Black bean gruel!"*
The Low-Down:
Children have an unlimited capacity to ask this question. It is, hands down, the question you'll be asked *<u>most</u>* *frequently* as a parent.

CHAPTER 20:

The Last Word

I'm honoured you chose to spend some time reading this book and I hope you're feeling confident as a momma right now.

This book takes you to your baby's third birthday, and what a whirlwind those first three years can be. The early parts of parenthood—new motherhood—are unlike the rest.

In those first three years, your relationship with your baby is at its most *intense,* but also at its *simplest*.

The *love* is intense.

Your baby has a bottomless need for you:

"Where are you?"

"You're back!"

"Look at me! Are you watching? Did you see what I did?"

He isn't interested in what you might know or what you can do—he just craves *you*. He wants your acknowledgment.

The love is also *simple*.

It's unfiltered and uncomplicated. It's the pure adoration that children feel before they notice the cracks that make their parents flawed and human.

And your *life* is intense, but also simple.

Some parts of the baby years feel bogged down by repetitive tasks. Wipe high chair. Wipe bum. Wipe tears. Repeat. There's always something. You're always busy.

But there's also the delightful simplicity of days filled with toys and tricycles and outings to the zoo. And the peace of mind that comes with knowing that you're in charge of everything: the clothing, the diet, the activities, the relationships, the rules.

You *know* your child. You really get him. You're in it fully.

You're in it fully, until you're not.

The immersive fog that engulfs parents of young children begins to lift around the age of three. As your baby grows into a walking, talking preschooler, you may find, as many parents do, that everything becomes easier.

You can start reasoning with your child. You can ease up your vigilance around breakable objects. You spend less time on the bedtime routine. Your life stops revolving around the next snack.

You're not there all the time. The first unparented playdate or birthday party arrives, and then the next, and suddenly you're never invited. As he does more, you do less, which is the normal way of the world.

You lose that new-mom, or new-dad sheen. You become a family with kids.

Once your baby turns three, you've made it through the all-consuming first bit of parenthood that reorders your life completely.

You don't have all the answers, but you have a lot of experience.

You've got it from here.

RESOURCES USED & RECOMMENDED

Here is a list of authors whose work and ideas have been invaluable to me over the years. Some of their ideas have been woven into this book, although, of course, this does not mean they would necessarily agree with my interpretations and thoughts. All of these resources are pretty awesome. I recommend you check them out!

Guide to creating a birthing plan:

- ✓ "No more birth shaming," by Leah McLaren (*The Globe and Mail*: August 26, 2016) theglobeandmail.com/life/parenting/leah-mclaren-birth-shaming-is-about-controlling-women-not-protecting-babies/article31550367/

Pregnancy loss:

- ✓ *The Seed: How the Feminist Movement Fails Infertile Women*, by Alexandra Kimball

Baby remarkable:

- ✓ *My Own Blood: A Memoir*, by Ashley Bristowe

- ✓ *The Boy in the Moon: A father's search for his disabled son*, by Ian Brown, won the RBC Taylor Prize for literary nonfiction

Breastfeeding:

- ✓ *The Womanly Art of Breastfeeding,* 8th edition, by Diane Wiessinger, Diana West, and Teresa Pitman
- ✓ *How Weaning Happens,* by Diane Bengson
- ✓ *Biological Nurturing: Instinctual Breastfeeding*, by Suzanne Colson
- ✓ *The Nursing Mother's Guide to Weaning,* by Kathleen Huggins and Linda Ziedrich
- ✓ *Adventures in Tandem Nursing: Breastfeeding During Pregnancy and Beyond*, by Hilary Flower
- ✓ *Breastfeeding Made Simple: Seven Natural Laws for Nursing Mothers*, by Nancy Mohrbacher and Kathleen Kendall-Tackett
- ✓ *Dr. Jack Newman's Guide to Breastfeeding*, by Dr. Jack Newman and Teresa Pitman
- ✓ ibconline.ca/ (International Breastfeeding Centre created by Dr. Jack Newman)
- ✓ kellymom.com
- ✓ llli.org/resources/ La Leche League International
- ✓ lllc.ca/ La Leche League Canada
- ✓ breastfeedingbasics.com/articles/public-nursing
- ✓ nancymohrbacher.com (where you can download the Breastfeeding Solution App)
- ✓ bornandfed.com
- ✓ "No, You're Not Pregnant and Simultaneously PMSing, You Just Weaned a Toddler," by Tracy Moore (Jezebel: August 23, 2012) jezebel.com/

no-you-re-not-pregnant-and-simultaneously-pmsing-you-5937022 (Sample of her perceptive writing genius: "I would have bet money on Aunt Flo busting down the door with a machete within three days; bitch never showed.")

Sleep:

- ✓ *Healthy Sleep Habits, Happy Child,* by Marc Weissbluth, M.D.
- ✓ *Why We Sleep: Unlocking the Power of Sleep and Dreams,* by Matthew Walker, PhD (essential reading for every human who wants to live as long and well as possible)
- ✓ *Sweet Sleep: Nighttime and Naptime Strategies for the Breastfeeding Family,* by Diane Wiessinger, Diana West, Linda J. Smith, and Teresa Pitman (particularly indispensable for bed-sharing with baby)
- ✓ sleepfoundation.org
- ✓ todaysparent.com/baby/baby-sleep/youre-not-evil-if-you-sleep-train-your-baby/

The evening fussies:

- ✓ *The Happiest Baby on the Block,* by Harvey Karp
- ✓ *Healthy Sleep Habits, Happy Child,* by Marc Weissbluth, M.D.

Solid foods:

- ✓ *The Omnivore's Dilemma,* by Michael Pollan
- ✓ *In Defense of Food: An Eater's Manifesto,* by Michael Pollan
- ✓ *Food Rules: An Eater's Manual,* by Michael Pollan
- ✓ *Baby-Led Weaning: The Essential Guide to Introducing Solid Foods—And Helping Your Baby to Grow Up a Happy and Confident Eater,* by Gill Rapley and Tracey Murkett

- ✓ *Child of Mine, Feeding with Love and Good Sense*, by Ellyn Satter. See also: ellynsatterinstitute.org
- ✓ "Timing of introduction of allergenic solids for infants at high risk," Canadian Paediatric Society, Posted: January 24, 2019, cps.ca/en/documents/position/allergenic-solids
- ✓ Any *Calvin and Hobbes* anthology or collection, by Bill Watterson (for a comical perspective on how nothing you prepare, ever, will appear edible to a child)

Discipline:

- ✓ *Discipline Without Distress: 135 Tools for Raising Caring, Responsible Children Without Time-Out, Spanking, Punishment or Bribery,* by Judy Arnall
- ✓ *Kids Are Worth It! Raising Resilient, Responsible, Compassionate Kids,* by Barbara Coloroso
- ✓ *Siblings Without Rivalry: How To Help Your Children Live Together So You Can Live Too,* by Adele Faber and Elaine Mazlish
- ✓ *How to Talk So Kids Will Listen & Listen So Kids Will Talk,* by Adele Faber and Elaine Mazlish
- ✓ *The Whole Brain Child,* by Daniel J. Siegel and Tina Payne Bryson

Parenting guides:

- ✓ *Kids These days: A Game Plan for (Re) Connecting with Those We Teach, Lead, & Love,* by Jody Carrington (absolutely amazing! and she's also an inspiring public speaker)
- ✓ *Battle Hymn of the Tiger Mother,* by Amy Chua (a classic, and an entertaining reminder that children truly can thrive with all sorts of parenting approaches)

- ✓ *The Gardener and the Carpenter,* by Alison Gopnik
- ✓ *Under Pressure: Rescuing Our Children from the Culture of Hyper-Parenting*, by Carl Honoré (2008)
- ✓ "How Feminism Begat Intensive Mothering," by Belinda Luscombe (*Time*: May 10, 2012). ideas.time.com/2012/05/10/how-feminism-begat-intensive-mothering/#ixzz1xLzgckOw
- ✓ *How To Raise An Adult: Break Free of the Overparenting Trap and Prepare Your Kids for Success,* by Julie Lythcott-Haims
- ✓ "The Over-Parenting Trap: How to Avoid 'Checklisted' Childhoods and Raise Adults," by Julie Lythcott-Haims (Time: June 9, 2015), time.com/3910020/the-over-parenting-trap-how-to-avoid-checklisted-childhoods-and-raise-adults/
- ✓ "Attachment parenting has been taken to the extreme. Here's my case for semi-detached," by Leah McLaren (*The Globe and Mail*: May 22, 2014), theglobeandmail.com/life/parenting/a-guide-to-semi-detached-parenting/article18809304/
- ✓ *Hold On to Your Kids: Why Parents Need to Matter More Than Peers*, by Gordon Neufeld and Gabor Maté
- ✓ "Confessions of an accidental attachment parent," by Susanna Schrobsdorff (*Time*: May 10, 2012), ideas.time.com/2012/05/10/confessions-of-an-accidental-attachment-parent/#ixzz1xM0OahtF (*I love, love this short article!*)

How-to-stop-yelling at-your-kids *FREE* e-course:

- ✓ sarahrosensweet.com/ (excellent online resource on how to get your kids to follow the limits you set, without yelling, from a renowned, Toronto-based parenting coach)

Outdoor play:

- *Let Them Eat Dirt: How Microbes Can Make Your Child Healthier* by B. Brett Finlay and Marie-Claire Arrieta
- *Playborhood: Turn Your Neighborhood into a Place for Play*, by Mike Lanza
- ActiveForLife.com another great source of ideas
- OutsidePLAY.ca is a Canadian-made, online, *risk-assessment tool* for parents and caregivers
- playborhood.com has inspiring stories of innovative communities throughout the US and Canada that have successfully created vibrant neighbourhood play lives for their children
- freerangekids.com/ makes the case that children deserve some unsupervised time
- letgrow.org more resources for nurturing play-friendly communities
- youtube.com/watch?v=Bg-GEzM7iTk TED Talk: Dr. Peter Gray on the decline of play and increase in narcissism
- "Don't tell me my kids are better off bored all summer," by Leah McLaren (The Globe and Mail: July 7, 2016), theglobeandmail.com/life/parenting/back-to-school/leah-mclaren-dont-tell-me-my-kids-are-better-off-bored/article30788933/
- parkprescriptions.ca, PaRx, a prescription for nature
- child-encyclopedia.com/outdoor-play Encyclopedia on Early Childhood Development

Screen time:

- "Position Statement: Screen time and preschool children: Promoting health and development in a digital world," Posted

November 24, 2022, Canadian Paediatric Society, cps.ca/en/documents/position/screen-time-and-preschool-children

- ✓ See also: caringforkids.cps.ca/handouts/behavior-and-development/screen-time-and-young-children, which provides information for parents from Canada's paediatricians (Canadian Paediatric Society)
- ✓ *Technology, children, and learning: a handbook for parents and teachers.* University of Calgary. explore.ucalgary.ca/technology-children-learning-handbook-parents-teachers?utm_source=UToday&utm_medium=Email&utm_campaign=NAP-DigitalWorld (free e-book)
- ✓ *The Tech-Wise Family: Everyday Steps for Putting Technology in Its Proper Place*, by Andy Crouch
- ✓ *Reset Your Child's Brain*, by Dr. Victoria Dunckley
- ✓ *Wish I Were Here: Boredom and the Interface*, by Mark Kingwell
- ✓ *Hardwired: How Our Instincts to Be Healthy are Making Us Sick*, by Robert S. Barrett and Louis Hugo Francescutti
- ✓ *The Big Disconnect: Protecting Childhood and Family Relationships in the Digital Age*, by Catherine Steiner-Adair

Immunization:

- ✓ thepharmafist.com/vaccines/, a fun and no-nonsense blog post written by Olivier Bernard, part of his blog series, "The Pharmafist: Bringing life to science…and death to pseudo-science"

Sexual health:

- ✓ teachingsexualhealth.ca
- ✓ birdsandbeesandkids.com

Skin health:

- ✓ "A Guide to Putting Sunscreen on Kids," Julie Crawford, *The Globe and Mail*, published July 31, 2018, theglobeandmail.com/life/first-person/article-how-to-put-sunscreen-on-kids-my-13-step-guide/ (*Absolutely hilarious!*)
- ✓ *Beyond Soap: The Real Truth about What you Are Doing to Your Skin and How to Fix It for a Beautiful, Healthy Glow*, by Dr. Sandy Skotnicki

I ♥ Science:

- ✓ healthyparentshealthychildren.ca
- ✓ *Cribsheet: A Data-Driven Guide to Better, More Relaxed Parenting, from Birth to Preschool*, by Emily Oster
- ✓ *Scientific Parenting: What Science Reveals About Parental Influence*, by Nicole Letourneau with Justin Joschko

Explaining why you feel an enveloping gloom at what should be the happiest time of your life:

- ✓ *The Happiness Curve: Why Life Gets Better After 50*, by Jonathan Rauch
- ✓ The National Library of Medicine and the National Center for Biotechnology Information has several counter-intuitive articles about studies showing that people who value happiness most are more likely to be depressed: pubmed.ncbi.nlm.nih.gov/25678736/

Dealing with stress:

- ✓ *Don't Sweat the Small Stuff…and it's all small stuff: Simple Ways to Keep the Little Things from Taking over Your Life*, by Richard Carlson

- ✓ *All I Really Need to Know I Learned in Kindergarten: Uncommon Thoughts on Common Things,* by Robert Fulghum (classic)

Avoiding abject poverty:

- ✓ *The Wealthy Barber: The Common Sense Guide to Becoming Financially Independent,* by David Chilton (an oldie but a goldie)
- ✓ *Keys to Financial Confidence: Unlock Your Best Life,* by Marika Stimac (straightforward and modern)

Some perennial favourite books for babies

- ✓ *Each Peach Pear Plum* by Janet and Allan Ahlberg
- ✓ *Peepo* by Janet and Allan Ahlberg
- ✓ *Hippos Go Berserk* by Sandra Boynton
- ✓ *Moo, Baa, La La La!* by Sandra Boynton
- ✓ *Barnyard Dance!* by Sandra Boynton
- ✓ *The Very Hungry Caterpillar* by Eric Carle
- ✓ *Brown Bear, Brown Bear, What Do You See?* by Bill Martin Jr, Eric Carle
- ✓ *I Went Walking* by Sue Williams
- ✓ *Goodnight Moon* by Margaret Wise Brown
- ✓ *Big Red Barn* by Margaret Wise Brown
- ✓ *Sheep in a Jeep* by Nancy Shaw

Some perennial favourite books for toddlers

- ✓ *Yes,* by Jez Alborough
- ✓ *Chuck's Band,* by Peggy Perry Anderson (so many rhymes)!
- ✓ *Mr. Gumpy's Outing,* by John Burningham (beautiful plot)

- ✓ *From Head to Toe*, by Eric Carle (best action book ever)
- ✓ *Five Little Monkeys Jumping on the Bed*, and related books in this series, by Eileen Christelow
- ✓ *The Snail and the Whale*, by Julia Donaldson (full-blown drama)
- ✓ *Bark, George* by Jules Feiffer (fun sounds)
- ✓ *Roslyn Rutabaga and the Biggest Hole on Earth,* by Mary-Louise Gay (best dad book ever)
- ✓ *To Market, To Market*, by Anne Miranda (fun twist on a classic)
- ✓ *Murmel, Murmel, Murmel* and *The Paper Bag Princess* and *Thomas' Snowsuit*, all by Robert Munsch (surreal and fun)
- ✓ *Oliver Finds His Way*, by Denise Root (your two-year-old will be able to "read" along with you when you get to the critical part near the end of this book where the plot really thickens)
- ✓ *We're Going on a Bear Hunt*, by Michael Rosen (best repetition sounds ever)
- ✓ *Where the Wild Things Are, In the Night Kitchen*, and *Outside Over There*, all by Maurice Sendak (all classic horror stories)
- ✓ *A Sick Day for Amos McGee*, by Philip C. Stead (cozy)
- ✓ *Knuffle Bunny: A Cautionary Tale*, by Mo Willems (another great dad book)

DEDICATION

To my mother
Maria Lewcio Ziemkiewicz Cicero Sava (1946—2005);
an actually pretty good momma

I miss you in lots of ways.

ACKNOWLEDGEMENTS:

I have a lot of people to thank, so I'd better get started.

Thank you to you, yes **you**, for buying this book and reading this book.

Thank you to everyone who takes the time to write a review in print, on Amazon, or on GoodReads. And to everyone who mentions my book over drinks, online, at a bus stop. A first-time author can't make it without the buzz created by word-of-mouth endorsements.

Thank you to the hundreds of mommas I connected with through La Leche League and my new-baby workshops. This is your book as much as mine. I wove your collective wisdom into this book.

My parenting journey wouldn't have been the same without the influence, insights and parenting stories of the Sava Sisters, Steve's Ski Team, and the Park Friends. Thank you, Sylvia and Sabina, for helping me hold onto the common-sense babycare wisdom of our Eastern European peasant roots. Thank you, Margo Irons, for not deserting our friendship when I brought a potty to Kimberley. And thank you, Park People—we met when we were almost young, and you made those years funny and you made those years fun.

Thank you to Jayne Hill, Aron Hill, Hessen Zoeller, Danielle Caffaro, Will Ferguson and Amanda Lovig Hagg for commenting on early drafts. You caught tracts of tediousness, errors of fact, exaggerations of opinion and clouds of obfuscation. *Grazie*!

I feel immense gratitude that Emily Donaldson, an editor with an impressive resume, agreed to work with an amateur. Emily, I handed you a Blackberry brick of material and you chipped, whittled and polished to the sleeker, slimmer iPhone of content within. I am in awe of your skills!

Kimberly Glyder—what a beautiful cover! I lit up like Christmas when I opened your email and first laid eyes on the comp. Thank you! You are talented.

Of course, I would be remiss if I didn't keep going and add more people to make it look like lots of people like me and want this book to sell like hotcakes. Thank you to so many wonderful folks in my wider circles of friends—the hockey and soccer moms and dads, the former co-workers, the musicians from old orchestras, the amazing community of parents I've met by being involved in the life of my children's schools, and the Calgarians, Edmontonians, Duck Lakers, Quebeckers, Ukrainians, Poles, Argentinians, Chileans and Australians I've shared a pint with along the way. Thank you for weighing in from around the world to vote on the cover and to tell me it was exciting and cool beans to do this (and not just conceited and delusional). I'm lucky to know so many nice people! You are awesome!

Taylor Swift, I'm deeply grateful for the five tickets you set aside for us for the Edmonton dates of The Eras Tour. (Hey, one can hope!)

Let's see, let's see… Who else do I have left to thank?

Stephen-my best friend, my soul mate, and my partner in parenting. You keep me grounded, as the saying goes. Thank you for everything.

And, finally, of course, thank you Nora, Robby, and Natalie, for tolerating the fact that you are being raised by wolves. Literally. And for being the most wonderful, most beloved, and most remarkable children that a momma could ever wish for. I love you.

I love you all.

WHAT CRITICS ARE SAYING:

"Modern parenting is a competitive, high stakes sport, and you're in it to win it. 'Mother of the Year?' Read this book, and then hell *yeah*, you are going to *nail* that trophy."

"Penetrating, amusing, and uniquely insightful."

"Honest answers to common babycare challenges. Doesn't overpromise. Refreshing."

"Sanctimonious, self-righteous, self-assuredly smug, and with a superiority complex *nonpareil*."

"Overbearing and pontificating. Written by the kind of momma who shows up at playgroup and appoints herself sheriff."

"You can't do that anymore. I thought we all agreed to stop sleep training back in 1997."

"What sort of flaming misogynist just flagrantly assumes that every mom wants to breastfeed?"

"A new babycare classic is born."

"Best. Baby book. Ever. Or top ten, easily."

ABOUT THE AUTHOR

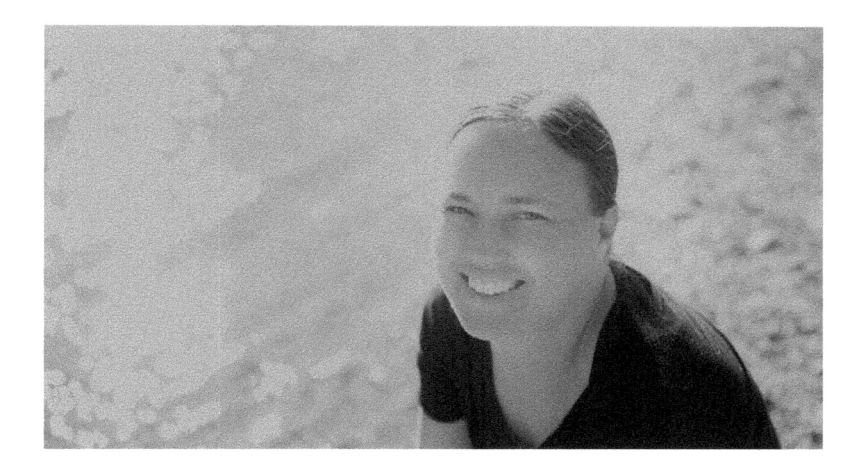

Susan Vukadinovic is a mother of three and a La Leche League Leader Alumna who lives in Calgary, Alberta, Canada. In 2022, Susan was a recipient of The Queen Elizabeth II's Platinum Jubilee Medal (Alberta), in recognition of her outstanding public service and dedication to education, children and community.